"Choice, moral agency, empowerment, 'patient-centered' care, user-run services, peer staff, recoveries! All so easily envisioned on paper, in mental health policies, and at conferences. As Myers shows us, doing the work to make these ideas happen in daily life is inestimably trying, unpredictable, unruly, and tumultuous for all concerned."

—Sue E. Estroff, University of North Carolina at Chapel Hill, author of *Making It Crazy: An Ethnography of Psychiatric Clients in an American Community*

"Well written and morally compelling, this rich ethnography details both the new promise of recovery from schizophrenia and its pitfalls in an American context. In the process, it explains how the experience of schizophrenia is shaped for so many by American values of individualism, independence, and work."

—Tanya M. Luhrmann, Stanford University, author of *Of Two Minds: An Anthropologist Looks at American Psychiatry*

"In public mental health, no term is more troubled and unsettled than recovery—and with the onset of 'managed behavioral care' matters are likely to get worse. But one of its versions, in one of its trial stagings, has been graced with an attentive chronicler. Neely Myers has captured the thrilling promise, rampant misunderstandings, mundane messiness, and institutional inertia occasioned (or exposed) by recovery. . . . This is public-interest ethnography with head and heart fiercely engaged."

—Kim Hopper, Nathan Kline Institute for Psychiatric Research, author of *Reckoning with Homelessness*

D0813328

RECOVERY'S EDGE

RECOVERY'S EDGE

{ AN ETHNOGRAPHY OF
MENTAL HEALTH CARE
AND MORAL AGENCY }

Neely Laurenzo Myers

VANDERBILT UNIVERSITY PRESS

NASHVILLE

This book is printed on acid-free paper.
Manufactured in the United States of America

Recipient of the Norman L. and Roselea J. Goldberg Prize from
Vanderbilt University Press for the best book in the area of medicine.

Library of Congress Cataloging-in-Publication Data on file

LC control number 2015010083
LC classification number RA790.55
Dewey class number 362.2'2—dc23

ISBN 978-0-8265-2079-1 (hardcover)
ISBN 978-0-8265-2080-7 (paperback)
ISBN 978-0-8265-2081-4 (ebook)

For Allen, and love

that knows no bounds

CONTENTS

ACKNOWLEDGMENTS

I must first thank my youngest brother, Joseph Laurenzo, for inspiring this book. He is a great artist, listener, comedian, and friend. When he was eight years old, he was placed by the state in a year-round residential treatment institution for children diagnosed with serious psychiatric disabilities. Bearing witness to his and my family's experiences with the chaotic mental health system of "care" inspires my work.

My mother, Patricia Laurenzo, has offered writing advice, editing, and encouragement at every stage. My father, Steven Laurenzo, has long modeled patient courage, stick-to-it-iveness, and faith. My older brother, Eric Laurenzo, and his wife, Shelly, have always opened their ears, hearts, and home. My in-laws, especially Nancy, Henry, Lisa, Mike, Terry, Tim, Joseph, Dan, and Vaidan, have supported this project from its earliest conception with good conversation and hard questions.

My life's work is made possible because others have learned how to experience recovery from serious emotional distress—and many have also struggled. There are people who are public about their experiences and people who are not. To those who are—Darby Penney, Oryx Cohen, David Oaks, Daniel Fisher, Pat Deegan, Fred Frese III, Elyn Saks, Leah Harris, Will Hall, and more—some of you are friends and some of you don't know I exist, but I thank you for all you have taught me while fighting the good fight.

Other teachers have also been invaluable. At Exeter, Douglas Rogers, George Mangan, and Michael Drummey taught me to write. Russell Weatherspoon and Robert Thompson fostered my faith. Corey Zimmerman and her mother, Alice, Shannon Powers (may she rest in peace) and her parents, Robert and Pamela, and

Jesson Alexander all helped me cope with my brother's increasingly challenging experiences and learn how to channel my despair into writing and service. Later, my professors at the University of Virginia, most notably Eve Danziger, Edith Turner, and George Mentore, breathed life into my intellectual orientation for this project and inspired me to become an anthropologist.

Tanya Luhrmann and Kim Hopper—both incredible scholars and people—have been extraordinary mentors throughout my graduate and postdoctoral years. I cannot thank them enough. They have inspired me with their own work and always believed in mine. Countless hours have been spent advising me personally and professionally; helping me to navigate the inner workings of fieldwork, academia, life-work balance, and publishing; and writing letters of support. I could never be who I am without them.

The Department of Comparative Human Development at the University of Chicago was an excellent home for me in my graduate years, and I am especially grateful to Janie Lardner, our department administrator; Beth Angell; Sydney Hans; and Bert Cohler—all excellent scholars and good people. Later intellectual support and funding came from mentors funded by the National Institutes of Health (Grant No. 5-T32-AT000052): Ann Taylor of the Center to Study Complementary and Alternative Therapies at the University of Virginia and Mary Ann Dutton of the Department of Psychiatry at Georgetown University, Mary Jane Alexander of the Nathan Kline Institute's Center to Study Recovery in Social Contexts (Grant No. P20 MH078188), and Michael T. Compton, now Chair of Psychiatry at Lenox Hill Hospital in New York. Carole Sargent of the Office of Scholarly Publications at Georgetown University and Barbara Miller of the Department of Anthropology and Director of the Institute for Global and International Studies at the Elliott School of International Affairs at the George Washington University also offered critical support as I sought publishers for this book.

My reviewer Jim Baumohl and another anonymous reviewer provided excellent critiques that shaped the final manuscript. But really, it was Michael Ames, my editor at Vanderbilt University Press, who made this book what it has become—going line-by-line through drafts, and seeing the book as a civil rights document from the start. Joell M. Smith-Borne has also been an excellent and supportive copyeditor, and I am so thankful for her careful attention to this text.

In no particular order, I also appreciate the encouragement, comments, and intellectual contributions of Sue Estroff, Barbara Belton, Lisa Dixon, Janis Jenkins, Rebecca Lester, Eileen Anderson-Fye, Mary-Jo Delvecchio Good, Byron Good, Nancy Scheper-Hughes, Daniel Lende, Helena Hansen, Anne Lovell, Tom Csordas, Paul Brodwin, Conerley Casey, John Lucy, Mara Buchbinder, Kenneth MacLeish, Mark Furlong, Christine Nutter, Johanne Eliacin, Elizabeth Nickrenz, Sara Lewis, Jennifer Hammer, T. David Brent, Beth Broussard, and the students in my Culture and Global Mental Health seminars at the George Washington University in Autumn 2012 and 2013. My colleagues at Southern Methodist University, especially Sunday Eiselt, Nia Parson, Carolyn Smith-Morris, Caroline Brettell, Victoria Lockwhood, and Ron Wetherington urged me to finish this book—always a help! And my department chair, Karen Lupo, tirelessly helped me secure the resources I needed to manage it all.

In addition, good friends provided relaxation and support throughout my fieldwork and writing period, including: Amy Horn, Andy Davis, Hallie Kushner, Lainie Goldwert, Pinky Hota, Brian Mulhall, Jennifer Brondyk, Leah Sumner, Jennifer Lynch, John Blaeuer, Maricruz Merino, and Elizabeth Byrd. Their refrain—when is your book coming out, again?—kept me hard at work.

I am also indebted to the multiple community-based service settings at Horizons: the numerous administrators, social workers, and staff who supported this project. They allowed me free range and asked nothing but constructive criticism in return. The people using services at Horizons, the members, were also incredibly welcoming, as you will see, and accepted me, with all of my imperfections, as one of their own.

Last, but not least, I am grateful to God for the love I have found in my lifetime and my own little family. During my fieldwork and the writing of this book, my best friend and husband,

Allen, and our precious border collie, Hunter, were constant companions. Allen—thank you for the ways you share your love—your music, your faith, your patience, and our children. Even my sweet girls, Lilliana and Madalyn, joined in the fun. Lilliana was in utero my last few months in the field, and Madalyn came a few years later. Both made the writing of this book possible with their wonder and joy—my little candles in the dark.

A NOTE ON CONTESTED TERMS

There are many contested ways to talk about people who use or have used mental health services (in no particular order):

Patients
Consumers
Users
Refusers
Mad people
Survivors
Ex-patients
C/S/Xers
Members
Clients
Participants
Peers

While trying to raise awareness of the identity politics of each of these terms, this book upholds local usages as thoroughly as possible—an ethnographic tradition.

ORIENTATION

Where did we come from? We came from nowhere.
We came from institutions. We came from the streets.
We were no one, but we had a desire to change our lives.

—*Ed Knight, Keynote, Alternatives
Conference, October 2006*

O kay, show of hands, how many people forgot their medications today?"

A few hands went up.

"Oh, you're lyin'," Vera said, shaking her head.

The audience erupted in laughter. Most had been prescribed daily medications to address psychiatric symptoms such as depression, anxiety, and psychosis.

"Now, let's get serious," she continued. "If you met me a couple of years ago, you would have seen me walking around like this : . ."

Vera hunched her shoulders and stared at the ground.

"Overmedicated, no self-esteem, no self-worth, and—even more so—afraid."

Many audience members nodded.

"Afraid that if I walked into a social service agency they wouldn't help me with what I needed. I was afraid to make a move one way—to go back to work. I was afraid for another hospitalization after several times of being in the hospital for four, five, six months. My life was really changing for the worse until I became empowered. And then, I realized that for my recovery it was more important to help others. . . . Many people try to help themselves, and then help others, but my road was different. I needed to help others."

Vera was once, she continued, an "unruly mental patient" staging protests at her nursing home. She had been leading advocacy efforts for the past decade, and ultimately became a peer provider at Horizons, an urban psychosocial rehabilitation organization that served more than six thousand mental health service users that they called "members" in the local metropolitan area.[1] With the support of Horizons, Vera recently had applied for and received a grant to run her own, peer-led treatment program, the Peer Empowerment Program—also known as PEP.[2]

On that particular day, Horizons CEO, Steve, had asked Vera to give a speech encouraging other members to seek organizational leadership roles. For Steve and the hundreds of members in the audience that day, Vera was an innovator, and a strong role model for recovery. PEP's radical, groundbreaking feature was that "peers" directed and offered the services—which Vera jested later, "let the lunatics run the asylum." Vera explained to the audience how peers shared many of the same extraordinary life experiences as the members, which she believed made them excellent mental health care providers for members.

"They, too, have been homeless, hospitalized, and alone."

Having peers direct one's care, advocates like Vera believed, was different from having the usual, college-educated "case managers" because "professionals" could never understand how it felt to receive a psychiatric diagnosis or experience symptoms. Peers, they argued, would be more willing to give a member control of their own lives because they had made their own choices and were now living "in recovery." They had taken charge of their own lives and found fulfillment.

Partners in Change

Isaac was one such peer who provided mental health services to others under Vera's leadership at PEP. Isaac was a middle-aged, African American war veteran who struggled with the "dual diagnoses" of alcoholism and schizophrenia. He had heard voices and experienced visions and thoughts inserted in his head that seemed foreign to him. Alcohol dulled his symptoms, and he became an alcoholic. During a low point, Isaac lost custody of his beloved child to his ex-wife and had to live in a nursing home. Then, one frigid night, Isaac escaped through a defunct fire exit and bought a bottle of Jack Daniels—his favorite.

Shortly after he began to drink, Isaac collapsed. He nearly froze to death. Fortunately, a passerby found him and called the police. After being hospitalized for frostbite and liver problems, he entered another residential treatment program for people with dual diagnoses of serious mental illness and substance abuse. Many people with serious psychiatric disabilities are offered these kinds of "revolving-door services," services that do not adequately help people recover and then open the door to let them back in again when they relapse.

Isaac continued to be a revolving-door mental health service user until he attended a workshop at Horizons led by Priscilla Ridgway.

"This woman changed my life," Isaac told me. "She saved me."

Priscilla Ridgway is the author of the popular guide *Pathways to Recovery* (2002). In the book, she described herself as "an accidental mystic, a person with a traumatic brain injury and someone who has struggled with depression and 'PTSD,'" which gave her "the gift of greater depth of awareness." After taking one of her classes at Horizons, Isaac was able to enter his own version of recovery. He stayed sober and eventually moved into his own apartment, regained some custody of his child, and engaged in part-time work at Horizons as a peer mental health service provider.

At one point during my research for this book, Isaac and I had the opportunity to see Priscilla Ridgway speak to a very large conference for peer leaders. She came on stage and began to speak but then stopped midsentence.

"Oh, my," she said, and put her hand to her mouth. "Excuse me, but I just saw someone I met several years ago in a workshop I was giving, and I am so amazed by the individual I am seeing. He has transformed, I can see, and this is a wonderful moment. Isaac, you look wonderful, and it's so moving to see you out there. Obviously, you are doing really well in your quest for recovery."

Isaac beamed.

"I am so thrilled," she said, wiping away tears, "that we sit here as equals today, partners in changing the lives of others."

What Is Recovery?

Isaac's story is not unusual. During the research for this book, I met many people who described themselves as "in recovery" from serious psychiatric diagnoses like schizophrenia and bipolar disorder. They typically repudiated a biomedical focus on diagnoses, symptoms, and functioning, which they considered demeaning. No one appreciates being called "low-functioning" or "sick" or being told that they have an illness "worse than cancer," they told me. I knew from my own experiences that this could be very frightening. When my own brother was first diagnosed with schizophrenia at a very young age, I had a terrible nightmare that he had swallowed nails. I knew they would tear him apart inside, and there was nothing I could do.

Our fear of a diagnosis of serious mental illness in American culture is very strong. The experience of mental illness can seriously disrupt a person's life narrative and our expectations for them. If this disruption continues unchecked, it can impair a person's sense that they can move forward, be accountable, and live a meaningful life.

However, when I asked people in recovery about their lives, they spoke in invigorating ways about their extraordinary experiences. They talked about "transformation" and "healing" from "serious emotional distress" (Deegan 2002; Fisher 1993). They had meaningful lives, jobs, and children. I met authors, artists, psychologists, psychiatrists, and lawyers, all contributing members of their home communities, all in recovery from serious mental illness.

In the research literature, "recovery" typically referred to a reduction in symptoms and a return to the life one might have been expected to lead if one had never become ill—or possibly even a better life. The Vermont Longitudinal Study, for example, showed that with some community-based supports, two-thirds of "chronic patients," continuously hospitalized for six years or more, could live independently in the community (Harding, Zubin, and Strauss 1987). At least one-third of study participants returned to the same kind of life they had lived before, if not a better life. In a complementary study, hospitalized patients who did not have positive supports had *worse* outcomes upon release into the community (DeSisto et al. 1995). Another review of ten studies of recovery found up to one-third of subjects achieving a full recovery (Davidson and McGlashan 1997:37). International research suggested similar findings, with some countries having higher rates of recovery than others, especially "non-Western" countries (Calabrese and Corrigan 2005; Hopper 2007b). Such accounts pose difficult questions—if recovery is possible, how can we better promote recovery?

People in recovery have been talking about this for decades. Increasingly, you can read intimate accounts of people's experiences of extreme mental states and restoration. Professor Gail Hornstein has compiled a list of first-person narratives of illness and recovery available on her website, now numbering 700+ references. In addition, numerous stories are on the MindFreedom (*www.mindfreedom.org*) and Schizophrenia.com websites. Some narratives I personally enjoyed included Bassman 2001; Beers 1960 [1908]; Deegan 1993; Fekete 2004; Fisher 1994; Henderson 2004; North 1987; Nudel 2009; Saks 2007; Schiller and Bennet 1996; Steele and Berman 2001; Tsai 2002; and Walsh 1996. And you can meet an increasing number of people in recovery— just attend their lectures and conferences, read their books, and watch their TED talks. I tried this myself because as a researcher I wanted to know how people managed to recover when so many others became caught in what is widely regarded to be a fragmented, inadequate, revolving-door mental health care system. And as a big sister, I wanted to know how to best help my brother.

Recovery advocates, I found, shared many of my questions. They demanded that the general public reconsider how best to handle mad experiences (Clay et al. 2005; Mead and Copeland 2000) and help people diagnosed with mental illnesses find meaning in life

(Copeland 2008; Ridgway et al. 2002). They envisioned recovery as a growth process (with room for setbacks) rather than the attainment of predetermined benchmarks. Recovered psychologist Deegan (2002), for example, described recovery as "a transformative process in which the old self is gradually let go of and a new sense of self emerges." In a similar vein, Anthony (2000:159) described recovery as a:

> deeply personal, unique process of changing one's attitudes, values, feelings, goals, skills, and/or roles. It's a way of living a satisfying, hopeful, and contributing life even within the limitations caused by the illness. Recovery involves the development of new meaning and purpose in one's life as one grows beyond the catastrophic effects of mental illness.

This definition resonated with another oft-used definition of recovery by Isaac's own Priscilla Ridgway:

> Recovery is a process, a way of life, and attitude, and a way of approaching the day's challenges. . . . The need is to meet the challenge of the disability and to reestablish a new and valued sense of integrity and purpose within and beyond the limits of the disability; the aspiration is to live, work, and love in a community in which one makes a significant contribution. (Ridgway et al., 2002:5)

Anyone could achieve recovery—a meaningful life and the ability to live, work, and love in the community—advocates claimed, with the right kind of recovery-oriented institutional support. Institutions could foster, for example, an attitude of hope, humor, mutual respect, humility, cooperation, trust, and love between service users and providers (Anthony 2000; Fisher and Chamberlin 2004; Mead and Copeland 2000). These were lofty goals, but there was energy behind the conviction that services could become more recovery-oriented. As evidence mounted that recovery was possible, recovery advocates—including clinicians, families, and peers—encouraged hope and action for people seeking recovery rather than despair and resignation (Deegan 2003; Fisher and Chamberlin 2004; Frese 1998; Ragins 2002).

As the turn of the millennium approached, demands for reform gained potency, and advocates' core concepts of empowerment, self-determination, and freedom of choice informed seemingly radical public recommendations for reform, such as President Bush's influential Presidential New Freedom Commission (Jacobson and Curtis 2000; PNFCMH 2003; SAMHSA 2006). Recovery advocates delivered concrete assistance, such as publishing and disseminating self-help programs and operating "technical assistance centers" for mad advocacy and peer services. They also staged protests, celebrations, and conferences around the globe, working tirelessly to demand more humane treatment (Chamberlin 1990; Cohen 2001; Jacobson 2004; Lewis 2006; Rissmiller and Rissmiller 2006).

I attended many of these events, looking for answers. And I found that, for the first time in two centuries, people diagnosed with serious mental illnesses were transgressing the highly contested social, moral, and legal boundaries that prevented them from having a voice in their own lives—transgressions that may have provoked their confinement in an earlier age (Goffman 1961). Their efforts—at times supported by family members, professionals, and other advocates (e.g., disability rights)—won them credibility with state and federal mental health policymakers and provoked proposals for recovery-oriented reform.

Recovery-Oriented Care

This naturally prompted the question—what would be the rules, roles, and relationships of a recovery-oriented mental health care system? An ethnographic perspective on state-level, recovery-related reform in Wisconsin is well-documented in another book and is not necessary here (Jacobson 2004). But based on the efforts of advocates and states like Wisconsin, in 2004, President Bush's *New Freedom Commission* recommended that the American mental health care system shift toward using recovery-oriented services. The commission's recommendations were unfunded, and states had to enact them on their own, but some—cue Horizons—would try.

In this moment, "recovery-oriented services" meant minimizing the seemingly toxic impacts of the traditional mental health system. The "traditional" mental health system, the commission found, did not offer enough independence, empowerment, and hope for service users to transform their everyday lives. The traditional model accentuated principles of rehabilitation: stabilize the illness, reduce the negative impacts of illness, and help clients avoid rehospitalization. In contrast, the so-called recovery model accentuated the positive (see Appendix I). It suggested that people's goals should include being reintegrated into a community of one's own choosing in a way that was meaningful to them. Recovery advocates also argued that a person with lived experience that provides services—a "peer"—might offer people the opportunity to try and fail, make mistakes, and learn from them, which many thought was what users most needed to recover.

Policymakers were perhaps also motivated by the imagined cost-savings of people living (and working) in recovery. Around this time, treating a "chronically ill" adult with severe mental illness cost an estimated average of $19,900 per year per person (Harwood 2000). If people with psychiatric disabilities could be put back to work and stop receiving social security disability incomes (albeit a meager stipend) and Medicaid (public health care insurance plans, not then standard in the United States), some thought they would pose less of a fiscal burden. A recovery-oriented mental health system, proponents argued, would produce citizens *in recovery* rather than expensive, chronic mental patients (Solomon and Stanhope 2004). But first, everyone needed to identify how the system would produce recovered public mental health service users.

Horizons administrators, guided by Steve, the new CEO, thus began to develop and implement an organizational philosophy of recovery-oriented care—a philosophy, I discovered, that was deeply informed by US cultural values and expectations. Part of Steve's plan was to involve peers like Vera—people in recovery—to spur the revolution from the ground up. He also had "shaken up" organizational leadership from the top-down. His new Director of Recovery, a peer named Melanie, had put together the event where Vera was speaking. Melanie openly disclosed her experiences as a "recovered" consumer-turned-PhD as part of her job description. He also asked Melanie to help Vera give a speech to the members that would motivate them to take charge of their own treatment plans, and let people know that the organization needed to head in a new direction for legitimate reform.

The "Center" of the Revolution

Back in the hotel ballroom where I watched Vera deliver her speech to hundreds of members (which was also the first place I personally met her), Vera explained her perception of the organizational change needed to promote recovery:

> There's some Horizons staff that don't really want to change. They don't want to give up the power and control. Staff needs to change. So I would like us to say together as leaders—we need your help! We need your help to change the behaviors and mentality of staff today! There are so many great ones and there are some who don't get it. To them, we need to say together: will everyone please stand together?

And as the crowd rose to its feet, she began to shout: "*RECOVERY! GET IT, GET OVER IT, OR GET OUT!!!* Take this back to the programs and the services and the case managers! Take it and run with it!"

To be a national exemplar, Vera told the members, Horizons needed to implement a recovery philosophy that handed the power over life decisions and organizational programming back to members. Steve and Melanie expected and wanted this to upset the status quo of the organization. Their strategy seemed to be working. As the members chanted, the Horizons staff present looked uncomfortable at best. They had helped escort the members to the off-site Expo on busses chartered for the occasion so that Medicaid could be billed for that day's "therapeutic" events and were not exactly willing participants. But Vera looked confident. She wanted to lead a revolution in care, and she knew that Steve and Melanie supported her.

The Science of Intimacy

I was in the audience that day to hear Vera's speech because Horizons had invited me to conduct research on their organizational change process. They hoped I would have a success story to share with other organizations about how to become more recovery-oriented. My goal was to understand how Horizons defined recovery, what the process of recovery required from staff and members each day, and what helped and hindered staff and members in the process of recovery. I chose to use anthropological methods, recently dubbed a "science of intimacy, of intimate connections," because I am an anthropologist, and ethnography is the perfect tool with which to address these questions (Saez, Kelly, and Brown 2014).

One defining aspect of anthropology is ethnographic fieldwork, and I stayed "in the field" almost three years. At the time of Vera's speech, I had been at Horizons for more than a year looking at other programs and attending meetings. Vera's speech was the most exciting recovery-oriented moment I had observed, and I immediately wanted to know more. I wanted to see how PEP promoted recovery and compare this effort to the rest of the organization's efforts. Vera enthusiastically invited me into her program, as well.

PEP was housed at Horizons Recovery Center (henceforth, the center) where Horizons' prized 40-year-old Riverside program, run by twenty-plus professional staff, struggled to coexist with PEP, Horizons' most radical ten-month-old program run by an average of five peer staff.

Riverside's professional staff had a college education and many held a master's degree in social work. Riverside also employed college or graduate-level interns in psychology and social work. On average, Riverside staff served (during my time there) up to 120 members when it was open during the normal working hours of nine to five on Monday through Friday. Only one Riverside staff member told me that they were a peer.

PEP staff often talked about how Riverside staff were not "real" experts; they just learned from books. PEP's staff, such as Isaac, Vera claimed, "were hired for their *life* expertise and *not* for their *educational* expertise." PEP staff typically had been hospitalized multiple times, were taking psychiatric medications, and had lived in a nursing home for people diagnosed with serious mental illnesses. Most did not have a college degree. They were not certified peer specialists, which was not a well-established possibility in the state at this time. PEP staff and its 40 to 120 members thus shared the experience of being diagnosed and treated within the traditional mental health care system. During my time at the center, Riverside sought to make their professionally-delivered services more recovery-oriented, while PEP attempted to formulate and provide recovery-oriented, peer-delivered services.

During this time, I engaged in ethnographic fieldwork from the members' perspective. I observed public and private interactions between staff and members, attended center-based classes for members, and ventured out into the community with members to enjoy a cup of coffee, take a walk, visit a food pantry or shelter, or play a softball game. I collected more than 150 audio taped interviews, and joined in a myriad of informal conversations. I also led three focus groups with approximately twenty-four randomly sampled staff members from various programs across the agency (e.g., program directors, case managers). Numerous institutional handouts, publications, emails, brochures, and manuals related to recovery produced by staff, members, and outside recovery-oriented trainers fill a filing cabinet in my office. These activities and materials enabled me to examine the nuances of everyday life for members and staff as they learned more about recovery.

Horizons members' lives revolved around being a member of Horizons, and the relationships, rules, and tasks of everyday life such membership entailed. People from the outside world who were not offering treatment to the members did not come into the center. The members I met interacted with few outsiders who were not staff members at one of the various services that housed, fed, and clothed them on the "institutional circuit" (Wiseman 1979). Very few members had a cell phone. If they did, it was prepaid and used only for brief conversations or emergencies. Email also was sent or received rarely. The Internet was not commonly available, and many members lacked computer skills.

Even so, members' everyday lives were absolutely shaped by mainstream US culture, and the broader social, moral, political, and economic aspects of everyday life affected them deeply, even though they had little opportunity to speak back to these influences. As Kleinman (1980:26) wrote, any health care system includes beliefs and patterns of behaviors governed by cultural rules. During my time at the center, the contested culture of clinical life at Horizons affected each person's experience of care, and reflected broader, cultural values.

In his moving ethnography of community psychiatry, Brodwin (2012) argued that there can be no doubt that people diagnosed with serious mental health conditions are among the "destitute sick" in this country, and that they deserve for us to "bear witness" to their everyday circumstances (Farmer 2003). In that spirit, the experiences relayed in this book not only represent my work at Horizons, they represent over a decade of my work in mental health clinics on the East Coast, the West Coast, the rural South, and the Midwest. This is no cautionary tale of isolated incidents, but a comprehensive look at one location in the behemoth US mental health system of "care" that speaks to the condition of the whole.

Most people agree that the American mental health system needs reform, but most people only see the lives of the "destitute sick" as though through a glass darkly. We need a clearer perspective to move forward. If recovery is a transformative process of cultivating the kind of life one may have expected to live (or perhaps even a better life) prior to their entry into mental health care, what does it take to bring one's recovery efforts to fruition? In this book, I will explain how careful ethnographic work has led me to think of recovery as a process of rebuilding moral agency.

Why Moral Agency?

When I say "moral" I am not referring to a broader ethical code, but rather, the local ways that people come to be recognized as "good" in their everyday lives (Luhrmann, 2001; Ware et al., 2007). Psychiatrist and anthropologist Arthur Kleinman's (1999a, 1999b) work has long indicated the importance of being recognized as "moral" or "good" in a "local moral world" as important for mental health and healing. Angela Garcia (2010), an anthropologist working among heroin-addicted families, has similarly pondered the role of intimate relationships in the process of being recognized as "good" in one local moral world, and how the complex entanglements of human desire for intimacy and the constraints and enablements of local moral worlds build and erode lives and relationships among her informants. Erika Blacksher (2002) uses the specific term *moral agency* to describe a person's freedom to aspire to a "good life" in a way that leads to intimate connections to others. Recovery advocates also often describe recovery from serious psychiatric disabilities in similar terms: the ability to live, love, and work in a community that values one's contribution (Anthony 2000)—a community, presumably, with which one can build much-desired, intimate connections. Moral agency, this book argues, is the oft-overlooked driver of recovery. It documents—intimately, and from the ground up—how moral agency, the ability to be recognized as a "good" person in a way that makes possible intimate connections to others—is so easily eroded by the ways in which we treat people with mental illness in this country, and what people in recovery from serious psychiatric disabilities might even preliminarily need to reverse and replenish this erosion and recover.

NO DIRECTION HOME

I am Vera, and I am bipolar, and I am in charge here.
Can you believe that? A mentally ill person in charge?
Finally, they let the lunatics run the asylum!

— *Vera, 2006, Director of PEP*

B efore there is recovery, there is life as usual. For many members
that I met, this life was fraught with harrowing social conditions. Resources to begin the recovery journey were almost nil for
people whose lives were excruciatingly stressful and who were particularly vulnerable to stress in the first place. For many, stress triggered psychiatric symptoms.

One stormy afternoon, a woman stumbled through the center's
broad doors. "I am so tired! I am so tired! I AM SO TIRED!!!" She
wailed. A crowd gathered to watch as she crutched across the slick,
concrete foyer. Puddles of water collected under her after each la-
bored move.

"Okay, now. It's all right now," Charlie said in a soothing bari-
tone. "Why don't you have a seat?"

Another member offered her paper towels. She lunged past
them both, and collapsed on a blue plastic couch. We encircled her,
unsure.

Another member began to chant: "You're just another number.
Oh, yeah, another one. You're just another number. It's a revolving
door, and you're just another number . . ."

Vera came into the foyer and gently asked everyone to leave. In
the hush that followed, I dawdled on the staircase, peering over the

rail. Vera knelt a few feet away from the couch and then approached on her hands and knees. When she reached the couch, she reached out her hands. To my relief, the woman reached back.

"We're gonna help you find some rest, if you let us," Vera promised, seating herself next to her on the couch. She opened her arms to embrace the woman, who sobbed on her chest. When she grew quiet again, Vera helped her back on to her crutches.

"Let's go talk," she said, "of your personal recovery. Of your new life, okay?" And after commanding people to find towels, food, water, and dry clothes, Vera led the woman to her office. Later on, Vera passed me in the hall, and I asked her how this interaction had ended.

Vera said she had just helped load the woman on an ambulance. "Her leg was infected—probably gangrene," she shuddered. After she got out of the hospital, Vera explained, PEP could pay to put her up in a cheap motel for one night. So, at least for that one night, she was covered. I nodded, feeling some solace in this tiny gesture of care.

"But Neely," Vera gripped my arm. Her eyes blazed. "I hope you're paying attention, because people treat their damn dogs better than this."

Re-institutionalization?

In his last act as president, Kennedy signed the Mental Retardation and Community Mental Health Centers Construction Act, or CMHCA (Foley 1975). The CMHCA ordered state and county hospitals and asylums to release mental patients not imminently dangerous to themselves or others for treatment in the community (Grob 1994; Shorter 1997). Ninety-two percent of the people who would have been in the hospital in 1955 were in the community in 1994 without the resources they needed (Torrey 1997). In the meantime, the homeless population on American streets swelled. Some of the members I met recalled a time when they were given ten dollars and a bus pass upon release from state facilities. Many rode the bus to the end of the line—and then what?

Deinstitutionalizing patients from hospitals and asylums and then dumping them into an unprepared community pressured people unaccustomed to taking care of themselves to subsist outside of the hospital on their own (Shorter 1997). Before deinstitutionalization, the state provided patients with food, shelter, clothing, and other basic needs inside hospital walls. After deinstitutionalization, in the absence of effective contingency plans, many deinstitutionalized mental patients became dispossessed people in dire need of low-income housing, mass transit, and employment that paid a living wage (Floersch 2002:28). Under these circumstances, it was difficult to distinguish them from the poor, exhausted, and crime-ridden underclass (Myrdal 1963).

After deinstitutionalization, Social Security Disability Insurance (SSDI) and Supplemental Security Income (SSI) attempted to meet those needs. Receipt of these benefits by Horizons members often (but not always) included government insurance coverage for mental health and physical health through Medicaid. A Horizons administrator introduced me to this complex system: SSDI and Medicare are "entitlements" based on how much a person has previously paid into the social security system; SSI and Medicaid are poverty programs that require a low income. One administrator estimated that 75 to 80 percent of Horizons members received Supplemental Security Income (SSI) and, thus, lived on $659 per month. These members lived $1338 below the annual national poverty level for 2009 (DHHS 2009). Members who found employment had money deducted from their SSI checks, which made them less interested in work.[1]

Social Security Disability Insurance (SSDI), an entitlement program, paid members benefits if they had contributed social security taxes for a certain number of quarters (depending on their age) or if they were declared disabled before the age of twenty-one. Only 20 percent of Horizons members qualified, although SSDI came with more incentives to work (Reno, Mashaw, and Gradison 1997). Even so, people who received SSDI and worked had lower-paying jobs for fewer hours per week and with a different employer than the jobs they had held prior to becoming SSDI recipients (Schecter 1997).

Moreover, people with full-time, competitive employment were unlikely to have good medical coverage. In one study of companies that employed people with psychiatric disabilities, 24 percent provided medical coverage, 8 percent provided any mental health coverage, and 20 percent provided sick leave (Cook 2006). Without medical insurance, members could not afford the expensive psychiatric medications some needed to stay well. A one-month prescription of 20 milligrams per day of the newer antipsychotic, Zyprexa, for example, cost Medicaid $700.52 per month in South Carolina in 2005 (Murphy 2005). This is just a one-month supply of a typical dose of one medication. It was safer, members explained, to stay underemployed and under the poverty level to maintain insurance coverage for costly prescriptions.

And so people with psychiatric disabilities using Medicaid generate revenue for psychosocial rehabilitation organizations like Horizons through "billable" mental health services. Lawmakers created the category of "psychiatric disability" to describe "anyone whose mental illness significantly interferes with the performance of major life activities, such as learning, thinking, communicating, and sleeping, among others" (CPR 1997). If a person did not have a treatable psychiatric disability, usually schizophrenia, bipolar disorder, or major depression, they could not become Horizons members because Horizons needed to bill the state department of health for services rendered to each member. People diagnosed with personality disorders were also not eligible for care because personality disorders are not considered to be treatable by the state.

As social services like Horizons emerged to provide for their care, members essentially became re-institutionalized in community-based services—a situation that Brodwin (2012) has previously described as "a hospital without walls."

Staff at the center typically welcomed new members for a "trial period." Staff explained that they would need to collect some personal information to "open them" as a new member, as though they were a bank account. Being "open" made members eligible for "billable" care. Horizons staff, licensed by the state, then provided billable care to the members. As a non-profit organization, Horizons paid their bills—everything from the building lease to staff salaries to supplies for the art room—by billing the state mental health department. The state mental health department then paid Horizons with federal and state monies set aside for Medicaid and mental health services. Much of the money intended to help people survive in the community thus went to the operating costs of organizations like Horizons.

Once they received disability incomes and services at Horizons, most members had little incentive to work. They learned to rely on the institutions of care that they were being asked to use, which offered them very little in terms of meaningful, life-building experiences. For members, this kind of life, Hopper (2003:5) has written, was fraught with the "terribly complicated" business of learning to survive on next to nothing.

At Horizons, there were members of all ages: people who had been in "the system" for long periods and others who had just been diagnosed. At least 70 percent of Horizons members and all PEP members were nomads on what has been called an "institutional circuit" of care (Wiseman 1979). At least one third of Americans diagnosed with schizophrenia, in general, utilized the "institutional circuit" for basic shelter (Warner 2004:191). While some people do choose to be homeless, many of the people I met had no choice (Lipsky 2010). They had no other place to go. In order to survive on meager incomes with few resources and little social support, people continually transitioned—monthly, daily, hourly—between institutions on the circuit. These included hospitals, jails, prisons, and inadequate community settings like shelters, nursing homes, outpatient day programs, and the streets (Hopper et al. 1997; Warner 2004).

The process of achieving recovery then prescribed by Horizons to these very same members, as I will explain, asked people to raise themselves out of this situation by becoming rational, autonomous, hard-working adults. Such expectations set a high bar for recovery considering the starting points from which many members had to begin.

Family Burdens

Where are the families in this scenario? Families are often the first contact for people who are in crisis, and many members explained to me the confusion and struggles of their own families with their mental illness. Most members had lost touch with their families after various kinds of problems—arguments over alcohol and drug habits, legal problems, homelessness, and so forth. Several reported family relationships strained by the member's intense need for money and care during active illness phases. Many also reported burning bridges with family and friends through "unacceptable" behaviors when symptoms—and tempers—flared. Some scholars have even argued that American families are more likely to socially abandon family members with schizophrenia than people living in other countries where recovery outcomes are better, such as India (Marrow and Luhrmann 2012).

A rancorous debate has long existed between family members who wanted the right to commit ill relatives back into a hospital setting against their will if they were being troublesome (known as involuntary commitment) and proponents of mad people's rights to decide for themselves when they need medical attention. I have read stories of husbands having wives committed for not behaving appropriately (Metzl 2010). I have met people who were hospitalized against their will and abused. And I have talked with a man who stabbed his father to death with a kitchen knife as a teenager because he thought his father was a demon. This man, now in his forties, wished he had been forced into treatment before his father died. More recently, the Virginia state senator Creigh Deeds' son, Gus, stabbed him ten times before committing suicide the morning after being denied a bed at psychiatric facilities because there were none open. Of this situation, the heartbroken father could only say, "It is clear the system failed. It's clear that it failed Gus. It killed Gus." (CBS, 60 minutes, aired January 26, 2014).

This is a very complicated issue and there are no easy answers. But despite such debates, the states' modern approach has been to reduce and empty inpatient psychiatric beds—and keep them empty (Rhodes 1991), as Senator Deeds experienced firsthand. Meanwhile, families struggle to support people as they experience round after round of symptom relapse and its associated setbacks.

Ronnie and his sister, for example, both shared their struggles with managing Ronnie's ongoing financial woes. Ronnie had a bachelor of science, a kind heart, and a cleft palate. His visible deformities, he told me, had prompted his decades-long trials with bipolar disorder and substance abuse.

Ronnie and I spent a fair amount of time helping him look for work. He explained that his cleft palate would keep him from being a cashier or a waiter, but at fifty-four years of age, he felt his back was too weak for hard labor. He had wrecked his finances with his drug habits and lived in an emergency YMCA shelter. He fretted about dying alone, which we sometimes made light of as we strolled outside with the nature group.

But then Ronnie died alone at the shelter. No one noticed for several hours. After his death, his sister wrote me:

> I can't stop thinking about him. I keep feeling somehow responsible, like if I had just sent him some money so he could live a healthier life, he would still be here. His life was so hard. But I was so afraid he would take the money and buy drugs. But there was no heroin or alcohol in his system when he died. So maybe I was wrong.

Ronnie's sister faced an all-too-common dilemma. At times, families refused to offer financial assistance, confused about what would be best.

Only a handful of members shared stories that included significant financial assistance from their families. A few mentioned haggling over inheritance money with siblings. A few lived with their mothers. Bella and Rose each had their own condominium, which liberated them from the rigors of homelessness when they were not in the hospital. Bella, a PEP staff member, lived in a condominium paid for by her parents. Rose had inherited her parents' place after they died, but she told me that it was in her siblings' names, and they "bugged [her] all the time" by painting the walls colors she did not like and refusing to let her boyfriend, Ralph, live with her.

Others were abandoned.

I asked Gary about his family as we sat at a table in the large dining room, sifting through broken toys. Gary searched trash-cans, dumpsters, and junk stores to find the toys. He showcased an impressive collection of Speak & Spells, remote-control cars, and robots. One, he pointed out, just needed a new wire; another, a new switch. After repairing them, he donated them to Toys for Tots and the Salvation Army.

"I always wanted to be a mechanic."

When drafted into military service, Gary became an air traffic controller. One Sunday morning in Vietnam, he had his first psychotic break. As we looked through the toys in need of repair, he described his experience:

> I was thinking so hard about the bombs on the planes, the atomic bombs. One afternoon, I was sitting in church and I started to—to disintegrate. First, I was aware of my body parts breaking down so I became a bunch of organs, then a bunch of cells, then I was aware of the molecules—the mitochondria and such—and then a trillion atoms. I was completely disintegrated and elated by my infiniteness until I realized I was the atoms—the atoms in the bomb. I was the end of the world. I tried to tell everyone that the end of the world is in us—it's me, it's you, it's us all.

Gary received a medical discharge. Back home in small town Iowa, Gary felt ostracized:

> For them, I was a complete disgrace. Where I lived, well, there was just a lake and one road around the lake. And you know that's all anyone ever went, around and around the lake, so they all knew. . . . My father, he handed me a bus pass and asked me to leave. At first, I was excited to get out of there, you know, make a line instead of a circle around that lake again—

Gary traced a circle in the air. "But he—my father—well, he told me not to call. He said I was dead to them. I died in the war." He scratched his head vigorously and redirected the conversation to his niece.

"She found me herself," he told me. She heard that he was an engineer and thought they must have a lot in common. He showed me cards she sent from a few years past. He was not sure where she was now, he admitted, and he hoped she was all right. But they had lost touch when he switched apartments, and to look for her, he would have to contact his brother who he felt had judged him harshly years before.

Horace also felt rejected by his family. After a major bus accident resulting in a serious spinal injury during a psychotic episode, his family sent him to a nursing home: "I spent a decade in that hell of [an area nursing home with a very negative reputation] because [my father] tricked me into going there. I was abused there, okay? They stuck a pencil in my nose while I was sleeping. They tortured me. Eight men in one small room! I cannot forgive him."

Months later, Horace showed me a card with a bus ticket in it for a Thanksgiving trip home. His father had written: "I am sorry. I am dying. Please come home."

Horace would not go. I tried to convince him, and he became very flustered.

"He beat me, too, okay?" He told me. "Back then, no one understood that I might have a mental illness, and he said I was a punk, and he punched me in the head. Told me to knock it off instead of trying to help me."

Tears spilled down his shaven cheeks. "I don't care if he is dying. He does not deserve to be forgiven."

Back to Work?

With tenuous ties to family, how else did the members subsist in the community? Some worked, which was a challenge. Symptoms were unpredictable; workplaces not so adaptive.

One afternoon, for example, Rhianna motioned me over to the reception desk in the center's bustling foyer. She was a member, as well as one of the center's part-time receptionists.

"Hi, Rhianna," I said, offering her my hand. "Are you feeling okay?"

Rhianna—usually very friendly—regarded me suspiciously, and then abruptly rose from behind the desk. She pulled me into a corner bathroom.

"Can I ask you a crazy question?" She used air quotes as she said "crazy."

"Okay."

"Did Jacob just walk in and flip me off?"

Jacob was the Director of Riverside, and I thought this unlikely. I walked over and glanced at the sign-in sheet on the front desk.

"No, Rhianna," I replied. "I don't think Jacob would ever do that to you. In fact, he is not even here today unless someone forgot to sign him in."

"Ohhhh," she sighed, patting herself on the chest. "Phew! What a relief! Sometimes I get these ideas that make me so anxious I can't concentrate. I just need a reality check, and then I'm fine."

When Rhianna worked outside of the center as a secretary, she did not tell her colleagues she had schizophrenia. "But then," she told me, "I might be sitting there at work and suddenly smell something burning. I had to ask if someone else smelled it, too, I mean, what if we were on fire? And, then, of course, there was no fire, and after a few rounds of this I would get fired for being disruptive."

Since Rhianna had not disclosed her illness up front, her employers could fire her. "But if you're honest up front, they just don't hire you, because they know if they fire you they can get sued if you use the ADA," she told me matter-of-factly. Other members reported having the same experience.

The ADA, or Americans with Disabilities Act (1990), is supposed to provide people with psychiatric disabilities "accommodations" to deter discrimination and enable them to remain in their jobs. Accommodations promoted by the ADA for psychiatric disabilities included flexible schedules, incentives to work, and training other staff to reduce stigma. To have a right to such accommodations, though, people had to disclose their disabilities to employers. Potential employers often did not hire users for competitive employment who disclosed their psychiatric disability (Farina et al. 1971; Link et al. 1997). In addition, 86 percent of people with psychiatric disabilities did not know how to secure special accommodations using this law (Granger 2000).

Curious, I asked Eric if he disclosed his psychiatric disability when he applied to work at a popular clothing store. "No," Eric said sheepishly. "[The store] supports employment programs for people with disabilities and has a partnership with Horizons, but I didn't tell them that I have a disability or go to Horizons."

"It seems like you were a good choice for them," I offered.

"I would like to think so," Eric sighed. "I have been there two years, and I am on the management track. As long as I don't screw up and bomb my work history, I should be okay."

A "bombed" work history meant breaks in one's work history, or "résumé gaps."

Eduardo, in his late thirties, told me, "If you have more than one résumé gap, they may not even interview you, and if they do, they are going to aggressively question you about the gaps."

He continued:

You just get your hopes up and then get your hopes dashed. . . .
I have a college degree. I got schizophrenia in my last year of
college and managed to finish. But every time I get sick, it takes
three to six months for me to go through the whole rigmarole of
going to the hospital, adjusting my medications, getting stable in
my relationships again, moving back into my place, and feeling
confident enough to look for a job again. And it's a Catch-22. If you
search for a job and find one, then you get stressed out; they may
not hire you. You have to decide whether or not to tell them. If
you tell them, then they can't just fire you any time because of the

ADA, so they are unlikely to hire you in the first place. If you don't tell them, then they can fire you if they find out. All of this stress could easily lead to a relapse. And then you're back at square one.

Some lied. A Horizons program director told me that he initially lied about his disability to secure his job in the 1980s. He made up a company that he worked for to mask a gap during a previous long hospitalization and prayed no one would check the reference. They did not. Years later, when he revealed the truth, his colleagues laughed at his ingenuity. "But that was extremely serendipitous, extremely risky, and probably pretty rare," he added.

At least half of adults with psychiatric disabilities consider themselves able to work, and the majority of mental health service users desired employment services and supports (Cook 2006). Indeed, members often discussed pursuing work and working. Even with assistance, though, one study found that only one in five participants diagnosed with schizophrenia secured work in competitive full-time employment. Less than 50 percent of people with schizophrenia worked at all (Gioia and Brekke 2003), and a recent study claimed that people with schizophrenia experience recent *un*employment rates ranging from 60 to 78 percent (McAlpine and Warner 2001). A complementary study showed that only 22 to 40 percent of people diagnosed with schizophrenia-related disorders were employed (Cook 2006). Societal stigma, low self-esteem, financial disincentives, and difficulty obtaining medical insurance all contributed to low employment rates. In the absence of work, many members spent most of their day at the center. At night and on the weekends, the best place to go was not as clear.

No Direction Home

During the day, Gary and Ronnie and many others called the center home. Staff and members were a kind of family. But at night, everyone had to leave. If people refused to go, a police officer escorted them out, and the building went dark.

One chilly evening, Ralph's eyes watered as he shouldered his backpack to leave. The shelter had given him a backpack to carry his belongings around during the day. Ralph hoped the backpack made him look like a student instead of a homeless person.

Hoping to cheer him, I lingered with him in the courtyard. Frank, a grizzled man in his sixties stood next to us. His cigarette smoke made plumes in the damp air.

"You don't know how it feels leaving here," Ralph sighed. "Walking the streets with all those people who are done with their day at work and are on their way home. Everyone is going somewhere, except you."

Frank tossed his cigarette on the ground and slapped Ralph on the back. "Hey, cheer up! At least you got a backpack!" He whooped. "So big deal, right? You got no job, no house, no car, no woman, no hope, no life, whatcha gonna do?"

"You're gonna keep on movin'," Ralph answered wearily.

"You're damn right!" Frank gripped Ralph's shoulders. "You're gonna keep on moving."

Frank, Ralph, and I walked on, telling jokes and swapping gossip and tidbits from the news. After a few blocks, I headed north. They didn't ask me where I was going. They knew I was going home. And that evening, as I watched people rush and sigh, grabbing a bottle of wine or some nice chocolate to eat after dinner, I wondered if they knew how lucky they were to be headed home, too.

The Shelter

Unlike me, Ralph was headed to a shelter. Frank walked him there because he had nothing better to do. Frank had the whole night to walk. He "slept off" his days at the center.

No one wanted to stay in the shelters, but there were limited choices for people without work or social security benefits. Ralph received public assistance—a check of about $147 each month while he waited for his benefits to be approved. If he used all of this money on a cheap hotel room, he may have been able to afford one week. Given the lack of affordable housing, even people who had disability checks (which were worth more like $500 per month) sometimes stayed in shelters to save money.

When I asked Ralph if I should try sleeping in a shelter to better understand the experience, he looked very concerned.

"You don't want to be in there with all those people. There are bad people who might try to hurt you! Shelters are full of felons fresh out of the pen."

"But what if I was in *your* shelter?"

He frowned. "I can't be responsible for protecting you."

Others voiced similar opinions. They described dark spaces ridden with danger and contagion: bugs, people with criminal records, thieves, pimps, and infectious diseases. They told me that there would be lines for everything—to enter, exit, take a shower, use the bathroom, obtain dinner, and receive a bed assignment. At one Catholic shelter I visited, everyone slept in two large, gender-segregated rooms housing one hundred people each beneath one tin roof. In the absence of ventilation, smells and sounds traveled well.

"Sometimes," Nicola explained, "it takes two or three hours for me to get in and get fed, then another two hours to get clean [take a shower]. Then it's eleven or twelve [p.m.] and I crash dead only to get yelled at around five thirty [a.m.] to grab my breakfast and get out."

Many shelter-users longed for rest.

"If the sounds and the smell and the worry didn't keep you awake," Nicola explained softly, "the fear would. Bad things can happen in the dark."

Most shelters let out between six and seven in the morning (some earlier), leaving people in a lurch. Most mental health programs like the center opened after nine thirty a.m. People like Nicola huddled together in the alleys, or near building vents that released warm air, or walked constantly to keep warm, having long ago exhausted the option of sitting at a local McDonald's for free.

Since no one could leave items at the shelter, people hauled their few belongings with them. The homeless could not keep more than they could carry. Nicola used a rolling suitcase to transport her few worldly goods—a seeming upgrade from the classic grocery cart.

Others preferred backpacks. They brought it all into the center in the morning, and they carried it away with them at night.

Sanctuary

For fifteen months, I watched them come in. They crossed the gated courtyard to our dilapidated mansion and passed through the towering front doors into the dark, windowless foyer. Most looked terrified, and we tried to engage them in conversation. What brought them in today? What did they hope to get from being here?

Sanctuary, I found, and the tiniest of creature comforts: a few hours of uninterrupted sleep, a few moments alone in a bathroom, or a warm meal to soothe a clenched gut. Others needed to fill a prescription, or wanted a person to talk them out of using crack again, a free telephone call, a place to dodge an abusive pimp, or a hot shower to wash away a month of grime. Most welcomed clean underwear, dry socks, and even cream to calm a yeast infection.

The newcomers paced, sat, stared. Sometimes they drifted off to sleep on a blue plastic couch in the foyer. Eventually, Vera appeared. Some cowered. Others hardened their eyes and clenched their jaws, preparing to campaign for their needs. And then Vera would offer the newcomer her hand and embrace them. She gave them a full-frontal hug—if they seemed comfortable—no matter their physical condition. And as she stepped back again, she would say, "Welcome home! This is your new home, and we want to be your family. We will give you love and respect if you show us love and respect. You will be able to do what you want as long as you act like you are in your own house and take care of the house."

She let them introduce themselves, and then introduced herself.

"Well, I am Vera, and I am bipolar, and I am in charge here. Can you believe that? A mentally ill person in charge? That's how it is here. No one tells us what to do. This is about your freedom of choice and your empowerment. We are going to give you the tools to change your life and make of it what you want it to be."

Next, she summoned the attention of others in the room and linked the person to another member, asking him or her to help the newcomer find food, or a bathroom, or a new winter coat in the clothing closet—whatever they needed.

"Take a nap if you need to," she told them. "Or watch TV. We aren't going to tell you what you need to do to recover. You are going to figure it out. And when you are ready, come find me, and we will make it so you can come here every day, okay?"

Some looked overwhelmed, frightened, and even suspicious, but many times I watched as their eyes brightened. Their humiliation, it seemed, began to lift in this moment of being treated like a person.

"Why was she so nice to me?" newcomers often wondered.

Other members often told initiates how she had walked in their shoes. She shared her history openly or members shared it for her. She, too, struggled with a major psychiatric diagnosis. As a teenager, she participated in criminal activities "to make ends meet" for her large family. This meant, the members said with pride, that Vera could name people's games faster than they could play them.

Vera showed me scars from burns and stabbings she had endured at the hands of her abusive, alcoholic father. He killed himself when she was a teen. After his death, she told me, she worked even harder. Then, early one morning when she was seventeen, Vera told me, she staggered into bed in the wee hours of the morning. Her mother came in and asked her to please stay awake with her. She told her she was on the edge and needed company, but Vera fell asleep. And when her hysterical younger sister awakened her a few hours later, she told me with tears dripping from her chin, "my mother—who I *loved*—was swinging from the kitchen rafters."

The priest helped them take her down. And then he gave her a proper burial. "He said—everyone knows her old man killed her with his violence and abuse and suicide. His memory killed her." Still, Vera never forgave herself for falling asleep. During the time that I knew her, she claimed to rarely sleep, tormented by the idea she might be abandoning someone in crisis.

One day, a sister of Vera's visiting the center told me that she was there to ask Vera to slow down and protect her health. Vera also had an autoimmune disorder, which at times left her exhausted. Her sisters begged her to slow down, she said, but Vera pushed on.

"My dream," Vera once told me, "is to really save someone."

"Vera," I said in surprise, "you save people every day."

"No," she said, "I mean really save them. To be there at the moment when a person is going to commit suicide and save their life. I have never had a chance to do that, and it's my dream. To save lives."

Over time, I grew to love Vera. I liked her so much that at times it was hard to maintain a critical stance. But I kept trying to separate myself from her agenda. And the people kept coming—in and out, out and in, an endless tide.

Ardella and Will stayed inside all day, but they also chose to sleep outside in the alley next to the center. They were both in their early twenties. Both had been in the foster care system. There are very few supports in place for youth as they "graduate" from foster care to help them transition into adulthood.

"We never had a sense of family," Ardella told me, "but we gonna be a family for this baby." She patted her belly where a basketball seemed to protrude from below her sweater. Many people told Ardella to move inside. She insisted the baby's existence required her to stay outside. "Shelters and programs for mamas want me and Will to sleep separate," she said emphatically, "and we need to be together. This baby needs us to be together."

One evening, I helped Vera bring out fresh cardboard and clean blankets for their makeshift home. PEP provided them with these supplies each evening to show solidarity. "And for the baby," Vera added. Ardella and Will used these materials to build a little lean-to between the back of the dumpster and the sidewall of the center. They proudly showed me their design to keep out the wind and maximize warmth. But after the neighbors complained, Riverside staff told them to stop sleeping in the alley, and they disappeared.

Months later, riding a bus home from the center, I looked up from my book to see Ardella and Will standing over me. They just wanted to say hello, Will said. They had found Jesus, and a new place to sleep, they announced, but Ardella had lost the baby.

And then it was my stop. I squeezed their hands and got off the bus, wishing I could invite them home for tea. My research was regulated by my university, however, which prevented me from inviting people into my house lest it seem coercive.

But I wanted to bring them in with all my heart. I wanted to let them all stay right there in my living room. I wanted to give them the keys when I went out of town. I even gave one young woman a key to my storage unit in the cold, dark bowels of my apartment building so that she could keep her things there (like a diploma from a very exclusive small liberal arts college). And when I realized she was sleeping there and doing her laundry in the building, I said nothing. Sanctuary: I needed there to be such a thing.

Late one February night, I stood outside in a negative twenty-degree wind chill waiting for a bus home. Even with a huge coat, and hat, gloves, and scarf, my body burned. My breath seared through my chest. Tears became icicles. After ten minutes, my fear of mortal danger overcame me, and I hailed a cab. Lucky for me, I had thirty dollars and a place to go.

As the cab rolled me home, I stared at mounds slumped in doorways. Someone's son is in that blanket, I thought. A half hour later, as I entered my building, a man huddled between an unlocked and locked door in the few available square feet of floor space. His eyes peered blearily through a slit between his scarf and hat. I ran inside to fetch him a woolen blanket.

In extremely cold weather, the police department mobilized homeless people to take shelter before the doors closed for the night, usually at six or seven p.m. For those who missed the deadline—or picked a shelter that was already full, and so on—the city operated four "warming centers" from eight p.m. to seven a.m. that served about a thousand people each night. At the warming center, people waited in line, came in, rested for an hour or so, had to leave, and returned to the end of the line. This constituted a brief moment of rest in a long winter's night—for some, perhaps not worth the effort made to obtain it.

That night, when I opened my apartment door, I gasped at the heat within (courtesy of my unruly radiators). I grabbed the blanket from the top of a closet, ran back out to the entryway, and gave it to the man, wishing I had the nerve to let him in. He nodded in thanks.

Back in my apartment, I sweated as I yanked off my snow boots and stripped off my heavy outerwear. Cursing, I hefted open the windows in a shower of flaking paint and set up my fan to cool my apartment down. And then I started to cry. What kind of world lets some people freeze to death outside while—at the exact same moment, a few yards away, but inside—the privileged are yanking open a window to cool down?

Cheap Hotels

If a person had a little money, he or she might rent a cheap hotel room. Cheap hotel rooms, at least in this urban area, cost $100 to $150 per week, which members could afford if they spent money on almost nothing else and had disability benefits. To get a sense of the hotels, I asked Monica if she would take me for a tour of her hotel room, typically called a single room occupancy, or SRO.

Monica was in her fifties and loved to wear vibrant colors. Her hair was shorn to her scalp to avoid lice, she told me. Around the center, she often sat with her arms folded under her pendulous breasts and rocked back and forth.

When I asked her for a tour, Monica looked at me as though she saw me for the first time. "You will not come at night, and you will not come alone," she said after a long pause. So we made a deal. Ralph and I would visit one morning together.

Monica met us at the entrance to her hotel, which I was shocked to find was located a few blocks from the center and just a few doors down from a trendy sports bar where my friends and I sometimes bought dollar cheeseburgers and watched a game.

"This is a nice neighborhood," I noted, as Ralph and I walked up to the entrance.

"Not in there," he said firmly, opening the door for me. The entryway was wreathed in smoke. Through a small doorway to my left, I spotted three poorly dressed old men sitting on wooden stools smoking and drinking cans of beer. A small piece of poster board hung next to the door. It said, "Beer served 2 AM to 10 AM."

I looked over at Ralph in confusion. "It's for the alcoholics," he whispered. "I bet they make a killing after the bars close."

We were right on time, and Monica appeared at the top of a long, narrow set of steps. She propped open a door to a dim, quiet hallway and let us in.

"It's so quiet!" I said.

"Yeah, that's why I said to come in the morning," she sighed. "They are all sleeping off their drugs now." The smell of stale sweat, cigarettes, and burning rubber (the odor of crack cocaine, Ralph told me later) hung heavily in the air. Dead cockroaches, used needles, and burnt foil littered the floor.

We passed a broken door on the right pockmarked with indentations as though beaten by a bat. There was no doorknob, the wood around the latch was splintered, and, Monica told us, "the light doesn't work."

"What is in there?" I asked.

"Oh, it's the bathroom," she said, meaning a shared bathroom. "I am terrified to go to the bathroom in there, so I pee in a cup and dump it out the window."

She would not shower there, either. "Asking to get raped is what that is," Monica shuddered. Instead, she took a shower at the center. At night, Monica claimed, prostitutes roamed the hallways. People piled into rooms getting high. Sounds of sex, laughter, and aggression permeated thinly insulated walls. Strangers tried to break down the door to either rob her or rape her, she said. She did not use drugs or prostitute herself, but these are the people with whom she could afford to live on her disability income.

Toward the end of the hall, Monica pulled her keys out of her hip pocket and unlocked the door. Envision Monica's room—a broken window patched with cardboard and duct tape, a sagging twin mattress on a peeling frame, a dresser with one actual drawer, nowhere to sit, no bathroom, no sink, no air conditioning. No way to clean a filthy carpet; dust flying with each step.

Her bed had little buckets on each leg. Each little bucket contained a viscous substance. "I put the legs of the bed in the buckets full of kerosene," she explained, "to stop the bugs from getting on the bed."

"The bugs?"

"You know, bed bugs," she told me.

A few weeks later, when I arrived at the center, Monica sat crying as she rocked in her chair. I asked her what was wrong, but she would not speak to me. Riverside staff told me that the heater in her apartment was not working, and that she had just been diagnosed with breast cancer. The temperatures this time of year were rather frigid, and the staff had decided to put her in a nursing home, but Monica did not want to go.

"Does she have a choice?" I asked her case manager, Elizabeth.

"Not this time," Elizabeth told me, shaking her head. "Not this time."

Nursing Homes

Another morning, I was sitting with Vlad reading haiku poems when Monica came up. I said I was sorry she was in a nursing home, and he told me that he liked living in a nursing home.

"Are you kidding? What?" I asked, thinking he was being funny. He was twenty-one years old.

Vlad nodded as he rocked himself in one of the business center's executive chairs.

"Sometimes, I really like living in a nursing home. What do I want to have to take care of all that stuff for? It's like having a butler, a maid, and a chauffeur."

A hint of a smile crossed his lips. Nursing home staff did his laundry, cleaned his room, made his meals, and escorted him in a van between the center, other appointments, and visits to his parents.

"It is funny, to help at my parents' nursing home," he said, "because I have to take time away from my nursing home to do it." He loved caring for his parents, he noted, but he could not live there due to the guest policy.

"But you don't *need* all of that," I pressed, "if you do your parents' laundry and make them dinner at *their* nursing home every weekend."

"So? It doesn't mean I want to do it for me, too."

"Well, what about a life?" I persisted. "Dates? Sex?"

"I can't bring anyone back to the nursing home with me, but the older ladies in the nursing home are often up for sex." He shrugged.

"Life is stress-free if you live in a nursing home. You just don't have much of a life."

$$\sim\!\!\sim\!\!/ \bullet \diagdown\!\!\sim$$

In January 2009, Vera took me into a nursing home for a brief visit. From the outside you would never guess there were a couple hundred people milling around unseen inside the old brick building on a wealthy, urban street glittering with fabulous people.

"This is it?" I asked as Vera stopped in front of an unmarked metal door and pressed a door buzzer.

"Yeah," she said. "No one can find the damn thing unless someone who has been there goes with them. It's like a speakeasy."

We laughed as a nurse appeared to let us into a windowless corridor lined with offices. She had to push the door hard against the fresh, deep snow on the ground and we helped her clear the way. Once inside, we passed several offices and came upon a locked door with a small pane of soundproof glass so we could see into the next corridor and the people there could see us.

A security guard smiled and swiped a card to let us in. At the end of another corridor stood a windowless door. The nurse slid a card through a swipe, and we passed into a surreal, cramped, pale green space. A dozen people shuffled aimlessly in front of a glassed-in nurses' station. Vera grasped my elbow and directed me to the right.

Through a narrow doorway, a hallway stretched before us lined with a long wooden bench and rectangular fluorescent ceiling lights. Every few feet open doors revealed tiny, sea-foam-green rooms crammed with two bunk beds, a large dresser with four drawers—one for each occupant—and a chair. Narrow windows faced the brick side of a building. I spotted no decorations, no carpets, few cozy comforts. And people with schizophrenia and other psychiatric disabilities stayed in these places for years—decades even. Nursing homes, mini-replicas of old asylum wards tucked into the forgotten hollows of the city, were the only long-term, affordable, stable option for many members. These were not fancy, fully staffed nursing homes with sophisticated elder care, but rather more like board and care facilities with a nurse or two to hand out medications. But the rules were strict—you could not leave without meeting certain criteria once you were there. And naturally, it was more lucrative to keep people there.

In a 2006 interview, Horizons' CEO, Steve, told me that housing the mentally ill in such nursing homes was "the shame of our state." More than half of the nursing care residents in this state had a mental illness. Medicare and Medicaid Acts passed in 1965 initially made sending users to nursing homes (rather than inpatient wards) more cost-effective for states paying for nursing home–based mental health care with federal funds (Goldman, Adams, and Taube 1983; Gronfein 1985). At the time, housing people with psychiatric disabilities in nursing homes reduced state spending on mental health care and kept inpatient hospitalization numbers low to improve public perception of the efficacy of community-based mental health care (Grob 1994).

While this state's department of mental health no longer received federal money for mentally ill people who lived in nursing homes, and the state paid about $100 per day per person who lived there, the use of nursing homes continued. One administrator explained that the political clout of the nursing home owners prevented change. Nursing home owners could lose a lot of money if policies changed, and they had a powerful lobby. Thus, the majority of mental health money continued to fund nursing home care even though more effective and cheaper care could arguably be provided in the community.

Members from nursing homes, like Vlad, arrived at the center by MediVan Monday through Friday and stayed from nine thirty a.m. to three thirty p.m. as part of their treatment plan. In the evenings, they went home and could eat dinner, shower, watch TV or smoke cigarettes, maybe place a phone call on one of the shared pay phones, read a book, or chat with other residents. Between eight a.m. and seven p.m. on the weekends, they could go anywhere they wanted but rarely had any money. The state garnished government disability benefits to pay for their room and board except for $7.00 per week (or $1 per day), which was all they had to buy cigarettes, clothes, shoes, and toiletries. Affording a movie ($7 matinees at the time), a small hamburger and small fries at McDonald's ($2 from the Dollar Menu), or even a bus pass (80 cents each way for the disabled) to attend a free community event was hard to manage.

Nursing home residents also forfeited basic civil rights as legal wards of nursing home personnel. Barry, a tattooed former biker in his fifties, told me over the course of several weeks about his perception that he had no voice in his own treatment. When he went into the nursing home, the doctors changed his medications—which were working perfectly well, he insisted—to medications that made him feel exhausted and ruined his appetite. Barry was emaciated.

"When I resist taking them," he explained, "they say I am being paranoid and tell me I had better take them or else."

"Are you being paranoid? Honestly?" I asked one afternoon in a group discussion.

"NO!" he looked angry. "I just– I don't– I shouldn't be a zombie all the time. I should want to eat. And I am over fifty! I have been sick for thirty years! I know what meds work for me; they just don't care!"

Other members nodded in understanding.

A few weeks later, Barry disappeared for six weeks. When he returned, he was furious. "Well, guess what happened?" He exclaimed as soon as he saw me.

"I was mouthing my meds and spitting them in the toilet, and they caught me and put me in the hospital as a punishment to make me take the medications!"[2]

Maybe Barry had a psychotic break after a few days without medications that landed him in the hospital, but he insisted this was not the case. He claimed he felt better than ever.

"I was EATING! I could eat because I wasn't so nauseated!"

In the hospital, he claimed, they continued refusing to change his medications.

"I just feel so oppressed, so powerless." Tears stained his sandpaper cheeks.

But, he added, he had decided to cooperate. To "graduate" from a nursing home, staff had to consensually agree one could live independently. Barry hoped he could make his own medication choices if he cooperated and graduated. After a year at the center, though, Barry was still in the nursing home.

When I asked him about his situation, he fumed. "Well, let's do the math. They get all my money so why would they discharge me?"

Was Barry being paranoid? Maybe. So I asked him again.

"You would be paranoid, too," he responded angrily, "if you had to live in a shithole like that and had to take the medications they give you even though they make you sick and you're constantly worried about every time you go outside because you're a skinny white guy in the ghetto."

Vlad also disappeared for nearly three months. When he came back, he reported that he and another girl from the nursing home were on the lam until the police caught up with them in another state. He seemed happy to be back. He missed his parents, and could not visit them as a nursing home escapee.

Where else to go? What else to do?

Incarcerated

There was another option. Some people committed trespassing or some other petty crime so that they could spend some time in jail. One-third of the inmates in Los Angeles County Jail have a mental illness, for example; this city was no exception. It was also not a good solution.

"Incarceration is not something that I hope anyone has to experience in this group," Randall announced at an All Agency Members' Council meeting.

"If you think free society treats you like something less than human . . . incarceration is ten times worse than being alive like that. My best advice to you all is to be working hard for your education."

Back at the center, Lindell told me he had been "in the pen" for dealing drugs. Lindell was in his late twenties, short and intense. He was the oldest of four children, he told me, and he never knew his father. In an interview, Lindell told me about his mistakes:

> I was a good kid but I couldn't see no way to help my mama. I needed to work! She was working three jobs and was barely alive. Even though I was smart and getting good grades I knew by the time I went through college and paid back my loans my mama would be dead from all her work. So I started seeing my friends show up with the gold chains, and the fancy rims, and the ladies, and I thought—hey I can deal drugs, too. I can do it better. And I can do it now.

After dealing illegal drugs for a few years, Lindell told me, he smoked a marijuana joint laced with PCP, "lost his mind," was arrested, and spent ten years in the pen.

"The problem is that the little man on the street corner selling the drugs is not the man making money. He is the man getting arrested."

Rosetta also discussed multiple incarcerations for trespassing and prostitution. "If you don't get caught, prostitution is great," she cackled. "You don't have to do anything and usually they'll get you high, so it don't bother you so much, and you got a body to keep you warm and a free bed to sleep in for a while."

Most people, though, hesitated to share their stories. To prompt conversations, I began to ask—which do you think is worse, prison or the psychiatric hospital? PEP staff member Joel taught the Dual Diagnosis Recovery Groups designed for members (the vast majority) who wanted to do a sobriety program that did not chastise them for being on psychiatric medications. He said that Alcoholics Anonymous and Narcotics Anonymous would often discourage people from taking their psychiatric medications. Some of the local groups, members told me, advised them that psychiatric medications were a crutch and they needed to leave them behind to be truly sober. As we sipped lattes at a Starbucks near the center one evening after work, I asked Joel about the difference between the hospital and the jail.

"On the psych ward," he said, "you lose your rights, the doctors have complete control and can force meds or restraints or isolation. You may never get out until they deem you cured, whereas in prison you have a sentence and that's it."

Joel stroked his beard.

"But in the pen," he coughed, and then leaned in to whisper. "You are going to be beaten and you are going to be raped and there is nothing you can do. Which would you prefer? Ya know? It's a tough call!"

When I asked Jamaica, she toyed with her rose-colored handkerchief and sighed. She explained that after twelve years in prison she had a sex change because being raped in prison made her "feel so much like a woman I decided to be one. Before that, I was very depressed. So I guess I found myself there in a sure way that I didn't have before. Sort of like a happy ending."

Many members had served time in jail or prison. Offenses included shoplifting, felony drug possession, drunk in public, disturbing the peace, trespassing, grand larceny, and even murder in the first degree. An estimated one in six male and one in three female prison detainees have a serious mental illness (Steadman et al. 2009), and over half of the prison population has at least one mental health concern like depression, anxiety, or psychosis (James and Glaze 2006). Despite these high numbers, only 40 percent of the mentally ill in US jails received treatment in the form of psychiatric medication, and psychotherapy is rare (Ditton 1999; Veysey et al. 1997).

Inadequate levels of care also followed released inmates into the community where less than half received mental health services (Veysey et al. 1997). This may explain why people with serious mental illness have a higher risk of reoffending if they have had a previous incarceration of less than three days (i.e., not enough time for people to realize they need mental health services), and a reduced risk of reoffending if their first appointment after incarceration is with outpatient mental health services, thereby connecting them to the treatment they need (Hawthorne et al. 2012). Experiencing homelessness or incarceration also increases the risk of experiencing the other (Greenberg and Rosenheck 2008), and many detainees are released to homelessness that came about as a function of their loss of employment, entitlements, or stable housing during their incarceration. US jails and prisons, many argue, have replaced the old state asylums as holding tanks for the mentally ill, and they are doing an even worse job of meeting the health needs of detainees.

~~~ • ~~~

DAVID CAME FROM JAIL ONE THURSDAY. He looked awful. On Friday, Vera got him a haircut and a shave. We gave him some clothes from the clothing closet. Then Vera took him to visit a clinic to get him a prescription for a heart medication that he needed.

Back at the center, prescription in hand and all cleaned up, he looked fantastic. I complimented him, and he beamed. With Vera's help, I was confident that he would be back to work in no time. David assured us that he would fill his prescription at a pharmacy over the weekend.

The prescription was still in his pocket unfilled, the police told us on Monday, when he died of heart failure. He also had a brochure for the center. They came by to see what we might know about his death. Vera looked bereft. "I knew he didn't have enough money to pay for that drug," she said, "but he wouldn't take handouts. Said I'd done enough and he'd figure it out himself."

The policeman asked her to contact his next of kin and produced a small silver lockbox they found in his backpack.

"Yeah, and look here, he had enough money." the officer said.

I watched as he extracted an envelope, carefully partitioned from the rest of the box. Inside, David had enough cash to pay for the medication that could have saved his life. But, the officer told us, the envelope was sealed when he opened the box.

He showed us the front of the envelope.

Scrawled in thick, black letters, the envelope said: "BUS FARE, TRIP HOME."

While the police waited, Vera called the emergency contact number David had given her. "His ex-wife," she told me with a look of chagrin.

Vera explained the situation calmly, and after some long pauses, she hung up the phone.

"David," she said quietly, "had promised his children a visit."

Becoming a "We"

Over time, I began to notice how new members adjusted to the center—a space beyond the rhythms of everyday life where people came to "get better," which we often referred to as "the inside" or "in here." *In here* served as a haven from stigma and misguided assumptions. *In here*, the members and peer staff had a psychiatric disability and helped each other cope.

I shared my struggles with nicotine addiction, and they helped me weather the withdrawal and side effects of the antidepressant I used to quit. In therapy groups, they invited me to participate, so I talked about other issues in my life, although I tried to keep it brief. As in a family, people looked out for each other.

On the advice of my academic advisors, I also began seeing an (outside) social work–trained counselor for the first time. It was important to experience mental health care, they suggested, and to have someone to help me manage some of the strong emotions that were bound to come up as I investigated this often sad and challenging topic, which was also very personally important to my family. As most members were also in some form of counseling, this was another experience we shared.

At times, I no longer felt like the members were separate from me. The members and I became part of a "we." Abu-Lughod (1986) and Rabinow (1977) might describe this as the development of "intersubjectivity" between us, an important part of any fieldwork experience. Other times, the social distance between us was staggering. I had so many more opportunities and resources.

At times, like Abu-Lughod (1986), I felt I was advancing some kind of persona because I was not always forthcoming about the comparatively posh conditions of my everyday life. This asymmetry made me feel less authentic at times, even though I never lied when asked.

I tried very hard to live as the members lived during the day. During my early days in the field, life was a labor of boredom. I went to therapy groups. I ate lunch in the cafeteria. I did not bring books or play games or read the paper, because the others rarely did those things. Days passed when no one seemed to have anything to say or when one person chattered incessantly about some droll topic.

There were some options. A darkened room with the most enormous large-screen television that I had ever seen at that time served those who needed to rest on the plush, red couches. The business center offered computers with Internet access, laptops with printers, free local telephones, a large boardroom-style meeting table, and a small library of paperbacks and magazines. A Riverside staff member even brought in the local paper and the *New York Times*. In the dining area, I could drink often ice-cold, truly disgusting coffee and stare out a vaulted window at the treetops.

Even so, many people were not doing much, which made me uneasy. I could watch the enormous TV, but the TV room was very dark. People did not speak, which I found unsettling. I could go to the windowless art room if it was open and had supplies. A peer support specialist named Bella was in charge of this space, and sometimes she told me long stories about her life or the lives of others, and sometimes the members chimed in. Many people had tremors that made art difficult (a common medication side effect). I tried drawing with my left hand to see how that might feel. We made many collages by cutting up magazines and pasting words and images onto poster board.

If I was lucky, someone wanted to talk or shoot pool. Occasionally, someone brought an instrument. But often the seconds dripped past. I regretted quitting smoking. Lots of people smoked, and going out front to have a cigarette seemed to break up their boredom. Eventually, I found the ability to join them without wanting one, but it took a while. When I practically ran home at the end of the day, desperate for some stimulation or relaxation, I felt sick with guilt. The others had nowhere to go.

One Foot Under

One afternoon, I sat with a newcomer named Azura when a member I knew well named Maison walked in. He had not been doing well, and I could tell he was riled up.

"Damn, girl! You used to work down on James Avenue. I remember you!" Maison shouted. "Lord, you look so different—so much better—so different, good Lord! Man, James Avenue! Now that's a place to be." Maison and I had talked about James Avenue before—the site of a notorious drugs and prostitution scene in the city.

"That's right," said Azura. "Hey, I am not ashamed of it. My life has taken many paths."

But Maison continued to look her up and down. "Damn, Lord, you look so much better!" Maison shouted again.

Azura nodded, thanked him, and then rose to her feet.

"I need a smoke," she whispered to me.

I followed her outside, noting her gaunt shoulders and golden-brown skin. She was a pretty girl, dressed well, not much older than me. We sat on the bench under the weeping willow tree.

"Yeah, I am twenty-eight," she said, sucking down a Virginia Slim 100, "and I have three kids." Her kids were in foster care in another state, she told me. She lost them because she was a heroin addict. "But I'm clean now," she added quickly, shivering. She only had a tank top on, and the wind whipped the willow tree around us.

Azura originally came to the center with another member, Bradley. Sometimes Azura talked wistfully about an estranged husband. Months slipped by, and then one day I heard some news—Azura was pregnant. Several staff mentioned to me that they thought she should have an abortion. Everyone was worried. Everyone was waiting, but Azura's pregnancy continued.

Azura seemed frightened too. She told me that she had some tough decisions to make. Bradley stopped coming to the center, and some whispered that he must be the father shirking his duties. But Azura told me that the idea of a fresh start appealed to her. She missed her children.

Then a man began to come to the center with Azura—a short, wiry, white man with a comb-over, wearing pastel polos, khakis, and a gold chain. He walked her in, and then followed her around the center all day, sitting in her classes, sitting next to her at lunch. Azura looked at us all in a way that made us realize she did not want us speaking to her in his presence. After a day or two, staff told him he had to wait outside. So he stayed right outside the gates smoking.

One day, as I was leaving, he stopped me. "I'm just Azura's dad," he said forcefully. "I want to make sure she's safe."

"You don't have to explain yourself to me," I told him.

"Yeah well, can I come back in? It's hot out here."

"Oh, well, that's not my decision," I told him.

"You don't work here?" he asked.

"No, I don't," I said. And then I avoided him.

Inside the building, Ralph stepped in to fill the role Bradley seemed to have had before. Ralph had children with an estranged wife, and he thought he could help Azura with the baby. He brought Azura her lunch tray and beverages and doted on her. But Ralph never spoke to the man outside. And when Azura went outside to smoke, she stepped outside the gate and her "dad" put his arm around her.

As we hung up clothes in a room designated for donated items, Ralph told me Azura had taken up with that man because he promised to take care of her. He gave her a private room to stay in and good food.

"And so, she sleeps with him for the room?" I asked.

"She wants that baby," he said firmly.

Staff gave up on the idea that Azura was going to have an abortion, and they enrolled her in a program for high-risk mothers. She was about seven months along. Then, all of a sudden, Azura disappeared. After a couple of months, Ralph finally agreed to tell me what happened. This was his version of the events.

Evidently, Bradley returned, and confronted Azura's "dad" one evening as they left the center. The man decided she was not worth a fight, and Azura lost her place to live. She took up with Bradley. They probably started using heroin again.

"Then she gave birth to a stillborn baby girl," he whispered. They had to bury the baby, but no one had any money and no one wanted to get into trouble. So Bradley, Azura, and Ralph did it themselves.

"You have to show me," I said, imagining saying a blessing over a tiny grave.

I parked on the side of the road. "She is over there," he said, pointing to a corner of a weed-ridden grocery store parking lot. Ralph gnawed on his knuckle. He was crying.

"We taped it shut. The shoebox. But we could only dig about a foot down. Of course, we did it late at night, and then we had a little service."

I froze, not wanting to get out of the car, not wanting to leave, unable to look.

"I'm sure the rats or the raccoons got her. Her grave was so shallow." Ralph sobbed. "She didn't even stand a chance."

Betwixt and Between

About ten weeks into my fieldwork, I began to wonder if I might be losing my mind. I had been crying uncontrollably for four days straight, which had never happened to me before. It was embarrassing, but the members and peers around me were supportive. A handful of long-time mental health care researchers warned me to be careful. This work wears you thin, they said. "It will leave you wizened," said the most experienced one of all.

When I shared my distress with my new counselor, she worried that there were no boundaries between the members and me. Boundaries from what? I wanted to shout. It was not the members who were stressing me out; it was the way society was treating them.

Around the same time, my outsider friends seemed increasingly fake to me—a perception they did not appreciate. I started to lecture them—they had no idea how lucky they were to have a roof, a new coat, and food. How could they blow $100 on a round of shots at a bar when people were digging in trashcans outside for food? How could anyone enjoy a hot shower when people were outside in freezing wind chills? How could I buy mascara when someone I knew did not even have shoelaces?

Even my husband, a friend of many years, seemed alien. I lay awake long after he had fallen asleep, agonizing over the softness of the down comforter and satin sheets we had received as wedding gifts. I tried sleeping on the floor, but I still had a warm dog to join me. I hated myself. It felt confusing to not really be a member, but to no longer feel comfortable with people outside the center, the people who—as I had just months before—lightheartedly ignored the members' suffering as the suffering of an alien "them." Oh, "those people." The strain of switching between these two worlds each day made my head and heart ache.

And then I helped another member move out of her apartment and into my storage space after her eviction. This would help her not lose all of her things. It was such a relief to do something. I decided to help the other members as much as I could.

There were a few member "volunteers" who hoped to gain staff positions eventually, so this was an existing social role for members, and I embraced it. Desperate to spend more time outside, I started a Nature Group with Ronnie. We visited the zoo and other nearby parks. I rallied people to play baseball and soccer. I worked in the kitchen making sheet cakes for birthday celebrations, washing dishes, and handing out lunches. I learned how to knit so that I had something to do when we sat around, and gave away each scarf because I felt guilty for buying yarn. I helped people look for jobs online and prepare applications. I attended consumer advocacy events and meetings.

In short, I began to act like someone in recovery. I felt so grateful that I had the capabilities to do so. I was not struggling with an unpredictable and serious mental illness, and people knew

I was not really a member, which meant I had greater access to resources. Moreover, I reminded myself that I had a project that I was deeply motivated to do.

As much as I wanted to know what it meant to be a "member," I began to accept that I could never actually be one. This was very lonely. But the members loved me anyways because I was kind and fun, and they were so desperate for what they called a "normal" friend, for hugs and gifts and stories about my weekend, for talk of my joy as my life took different turns, especially when I became pregnant with my first daughter. They craved the kind of intimacy that people offer others when they recognize them as a "good person," worthy of love and compassion.

When outsiders asked me if I was scared working with people diagnosed with mental illnesses all day (a top question), I told them I felt like Norm at Cheers.[3] The center was a place where everybody knew my name, and they were always glad I came. I—an Air Force brat, a child of nowhere—had never felt more at home.

And so "in here" eventually felt to me, as to many others, much safer, kinder, quieter, gentler, healthier, and more tolerant than "out there." We were creating, in retrospect, our own local moral world. In this world, we showed more patience and compassion toward each other than we received from strangers outside. Everyone gave what he or she could—physical labor, emotional support, and advice—when able. Money had little to do with our relationships; no one really had any, so there was little to compete over. But for some reason, we never translated our relationships to the world "out there." For one, my institution would not let me invite anyone in my research project into my home based on fears that it would be perceived as coercion. It was not just me, though; the members rarely met on the outside either. It was as though when we walked outside of the center, "we" ceased to exist.

Outsiders

On nice days, our eccentric crowd did occasionally spill out of the spiked gate into the community "out there," though. We held impromptu games of softball in the park, visited the riverfront and arboretum, and searched for better coffee at McDonald's or Starbuck's. We were an odd bunch—many ethnicities and ages, many secondhand clothes, many damaged teeth and ratty shoes.

People beyond the gates rarely interacted with the center's occupants. When they did, misunderstandings often occurred. One sunny day, for example, we lingered in the courtyard during a lull after lunch, soaking up the sunshine. The sidewalks thronged with pedestrians—a perfect opportunity for Morton to look at everyone's shoes.

Morton loved shoes. A towering man with a large scar across his forehead where he'd had a plate inserted after a wartime brain injury, Morton looked a great deal like Frankenstein's monster. As we stood there commenting on shoes, Morton suddenly shrieked in adoration and burst through the gate to tell a woman how much he loved her shoes. This badly upset her husband and pet Chihuahua. They never waited long enough to hear Morton's compliment, but the husband did call the center to complain.

Later in the spring, the members hosted an Open House (the first ever) to welcome the outside community, which I attended. Enterprising members set up kiosks to sell artwork, calendars, and buttons. The Riverside staff passed out pamphlets about the program in the Business Center. A handful of outsiders straggled in.

"I knew it!" One woman exclaimed victoriously, snatching up a handful of brochures on the mental health programs offered at the center and backing toward the door. "Dolores said she was just getting physical therapy here for her physical disability, but this place is for crazy people! I knew she was nuts!"

She dashed for the exit as several members watched in dismay.

"Wow, she's the one who needs help," Elizabeth, a Riverside staff member, said, putting out more brochures to replace the ones the woman had taken.

Despite our open house, relationships with the center's neighbors did not improve. Neighbors insisted the people they perceived as crazy and homeless should go elsewhere. They complained about people they spotted sleeping in the garden, on the roof, or in the alley after hours. They had property values to worry about, one man railed at Vera as she left the building to go home. No one wanted to be sipping a martini on their balcony and see a homeless person bundled below smoking cigarettes by the dumpster.

People stopped me, too. "What is this place? Some kind of halfway house?" they asked. I was never sure what to say.

"If only," Vera lamented, "there was a better place for them to go."

The instinctive rejection of members by "normal" outsiders deeply affected members' lives. Luhrmann (2007:151) talked about these kinds of experiences in the everyday lives of people with schizophrenia in the United States as "social defeat." She described social defeat as "an actual social encounter in which one person physically or symbolically loses to another one." The encounter, she continued, "must be contested, and the individual must experience loss." Despite the members' initiation into a mental health treatment program, the staff at Horizons could not change the members' impoverished appearances or the daily rejections of others. In a culture obsessed with vitality and success, the visibly poor and often tired members were regarded primarily as an unbecoming nuisance, and the terms on which they received "free" care were continually contested.

Even though it was our home, the center was a clinical space—a place for managing bodies. It is not a place to stop and settle, but a liminal space of supposed transition. It was also a place of "stuckness"; members became stuck there. They enjoyed the little bit of belonging they felt there because the outside world offered them even less. And that's why recovery, that "gospel of hope" as Hopper (2007:868) said, was constantly mobilized by Horizons (and policymakers, administrators, and mental health systems around the country) as a new language for making things right.

The Journey of Recovery / The Recovery Journey

During my time in the field, I heard many people describe the arduous process of recovery as a "journey," although they meant different things. First, the "journey" resonated with the American public's fondness for the romantic wanderer—a person who sets out on a journey to move beyond whatever defined one's life up to that moment (Bellah et al. 1996; Lovell 1997). In America, broadly speaking, journeys are a process of gaining perspective on the vastness and variety of life, finding one's own personal philosophy along the way, and then connecting in a mutually fulfilling way with like-minded others (Bellah et al. 1996).

Numerous examples of the romanticized wanderer appear among the heroes of American literature. "It's lovely to live on a raft," Twain (2002:131) wrote, in the voice of young Huckleberry Finn. "We had the sky up there, all speckled with stars." And who can forget Jack Kerouac's (2002) Beat generation treatise on the promise of travel: "somewhere along the line I knew there'd be girls, visions, everything; somewhere along the line the pearl would be handed to me."

As Ira Glass (1998) said on "Road Trip!," an episode of the popular National Public Radio Show *This American Life*, "You still—we all still—buy into the cliché about road trips. That what a road trip stands for is hope. Hope. That somewhere—anywhere—is better than here. That somewhere on the road, I will turn into the person I want to be. I'll turn into the person I believe I could be. That I am."

To embark upon such a journey was anticipated to help a person become capable of living a fulfilling life in a way that satisfied one's dreams and desires while mutually contributing to the lives of others. Unfortunately, instead of focusing on the hard work of repairing people's eroded sense of moral agency in the wake of a mental health crisis, the more common approach to the journey of recovery was to turn members into "billable" people with psychiatric disabilities, insist that they look for employment, and then fail to reintegrate them back into the mainstream community.

In my experience, the focus of Horizons' recovery model was work in place of wellness.

"Work is really the most important step in a person's recovery," Vera told me. "Members don't want to be dormant. They are looking for jobs. They saw somebody else get work, get a check, retire, and they think they can do it, too." Vera wanted to believe everyone could work, which she saw as the apex of recovery.

"There is not one of them that can't work. I see the future PEP as a training center where we promote working instead of symptom management. They know they can make it and we need to keep moving them up and out of the mental health system."

"Recovery-based" mental health policy directives like President Bush's New Freedom Commission agreed with Vera's perspective (and that of Horizons) that the ultimate goals for members should be to work, although all peer leaders did not adopt that perspective. "Most consumers," the Commission stated, "want the same things other people want: a sense of belonging, an adequate income, a way to get around, and a decent place to live. They aspire to build an acceptable identity for themselves and in the community at large" (DHHS 2003b:1). The resulting federal directives focused on promoting the idea that Americans with psychiatric disabilities needed to undergo "a process in which people [were] able to live, work, learn, and participate fully in their communities" by "living a self-determined life, maintaining self-esteem, and achieving meaningful roles in society" (DHHS 2003a:1). Over time it became clear that to become this kind of person, members would be expected to become hard-working, taxpaying adults.

In some ways, this made sense. One clear pathway to valued citizenship in the United States is to become a person who works hard (Bellah et al. 1996; Douglass 1992; Pangle 2007; Weber 1930). The ability to be productive through work is the moral foundation of the American social contract (Nussbaum 2006). It is *the way* out of dire social circumstances. As former slave turned "self-made man," Frederick Douglass (1992:560) famously advised: "Work! Work!! Work!!! Work!!!! The man who will get up will be helped up; and the man who will not get up will be allowed to stay down." Revered American founding father Benjamin Franklin also upheld labor as essential "for the good morals it preserves and the dignity and freedom for which it provides the foundation" (qtd. in Pangle 2007:27). Sociologist Max Weber (1930:111) similarly used Franklin's writings to argue that in the US, "the plain, middle-class man enjoys ethical approval in full measure." Work in America made possible the increase of individual prosperity, encouraged a virtuous lifestyle, enabled a person to contribute financially and interpersonally to the common good, and so generated moral agency.[4]

Unfortunately people with psychiatric disabilities, as I have demonstrated, were disincentivized to work and often could not find work even when they tried. Philosopher Michel Foucault (1965) once argued that the key transgression of people who experienced madness was an inability to work. Philosopher Martha Nussbaum (2006) also wrote that people with psychiatric disabilities have long been thought of as "moral leeches" because they took public funds and did not seem to give them back. It did not matter that it was extremely challenging to work given the social conditions surrounding psychiatric disabilities. "Free riders" in the United States were thought to keep the investments of good citizens from yielding their rightful return (Bellah et al. 1996:174).

In a March 2008 conversation, Horizons CEO Steve seemed to understand the cultural importance of work for Horizons members on their quest for recovery. "When you're talking about recovery," he said, "well, nothing says recovery like a job and a steady paycheck. . . . Employment is a huge marker of recovery—people are always asking each other, 'Where do you live and what do you do?' Employment comes with huge amounts of self-esteem, personal value and sense of worth, and connections to networks of people who can help you with things."

While all of this is true, as I have shown, at Horizons, it was also true that most members were barely making do. They were not ready to work and lived in dire conditions on disability incomes. Despite this, recovery in this setting (and in much of the United States) was billed as a "journey" toward work force re-entry. The journey so conceived required three steps: establish rationality, demonstrate an ability to act in one's own self-interest (for the greater good), and work hard. However, this prescription—a collision of good intentions and American cultural values formulated with little input from members—radically departed from the alternative journey of healing, growth, and personal transformation that recovery advocates initially articulated. Recovery so billed, I argue, framed as the *ends* of hard work access to intimate relationships via increased moral agency. Unfortunately, I found, intimacy was a *means* to recovery, and Horizons members would need supportive, intimate relationships much earlier in their journeys to succeed.

STEP ONE: TAKE
YOUR MEDICATIONS

3

To have a schizophrenic attack is the most awful
experience. I call it attacks because it—hits you [he
claps his hands]. And it goes away, and then you
can work on your bipolar. But you can't work on your
bipolar if you're having a problem with schizophrenic
attacks. That's the thing you take care of first.

—*Maison, Horizons member, 2004*

And so they tell us, "If you just take your Geodon, you
will rise to the mountaintop and get Abilified!" [Geodon
and Abilify are two antipsychotic medications.]

—*Amy Jones, Alternatives Conference 2006*

The first time I entered Horizons' boardroom it was packed with
people and mercilessly humid. I thought I was casually visiting
a community organization at the recommendation of a mentor, but
instead this was a turning point in my life. I would end up spending
the next three years focused on many of the people in that room
and their efforts.

As I searched for a seat, a man grabbed my attention. Everyone
else was wearing business casual, but he wore a baseball hat, a
t-shirt, gold chains, and sunglasses. He had lovely blue eyes. But
most startling to me were the jerking movements of his head—up

and back, like a horse against its reins. Simultaneously, his mouth grimaced and slackened as his tongue slipped out, in and around. Later, I learned that his long-term use of antipsychotic medications led to these irreversible, uncontrollable and chaotic head, neck, and facial movements known as Tardive Dyskinesia. Sometimes, they were barely perceptible. Other times, they were hard to watch. Stress made them worse.

I squashed myself into what seemed to be the last vacant seat next to a case manager I had met during a visit to one of Horizon's sites. She nodded in the man's direction and smirked.

"That's the show pony of recovery at Horizons," she whispered.

At lunch, as I selected a sandwich, she added, "Did you see him? Every time there is a recovery event, they trot him out and show him off."

After the conference, everyone there was invited to dinner at a fancy restaurant. Horizons picked up the tab. I came late, and headed to the end of the table to sit next to the "show pony." He looked glum.

"Hello!" I said.

"Why, hello, lovely lady," he responded, and jumped up to pull out my chair.

"What's your name?" I asked him.

"Maison," he said with a bow.

We pretended to be very fancy people throughout dinner, making each other laugh as we drank our beverages as though it were tea. Later, we busted each other sneaking outside for a smoke between dinner and dessert. I gave him one of my Black and Tan cigarillos, which he thought was delicious, and we talked about our favorite music. We had a great deal in common.

Maison worked as a Horizons recovery specialist giving talks around the city and state. He had a great apartment and the respect of other members. His apartment was a social hub. Everyone wanted to be near Maison for the same reason I did: Maison was in recovery. We all wanted to learn how he managed.

"Now," a staff member at his residence told me with a sigh, "he just needs to move out of here and live on his own!"

The advice Maison offered so fervently to others meant little to me at first. "You have to take your medications," he preached. "You must live it, learn it, love it, or you won't make it! And stay away from alcohol and drugs. They make your medications less effective, and your symptoms much, much worse." I prodded Maison for something more, but he insisted time and again—medications were the most important part of his recovery.

So, I began to visit him in his Horizons apartment. We shared his Kool Menthol cigarettes, fried chicken, and RC Cola. He never let me pay for anything. I came to the Music Group and watched him play keyboard and sing in a rich, bluesy voice. We took walks, and he showed me the best food pantries and the church where homeless people could have their feet washed. And then, one day, he told me his story.

"Schizophrenic Attacks"

As a young man, Maison left his impoverished New Orleans neighborhood to work as a nurse in the Korean War. Afterward, he settled down in a nice neighborhood with a wife and two daughters. Always a person of emotional depths and heights, Maison told me, it was around this time that he began to swing more dramatically between the two as the pressures of his daily life mounted.

And then, early one morning while walking his dog, Maison saw a UFO taking in water over the river. "It was absolutely incredible," he told me, "and no one can tell me it wasn't real. I know it was real! My dog was barking, too!"

Despite the years gone by, Maison still struggled to explain this event to me—an event that doctors later identified as his first "psychotic break." A psychotic break is a complete break with reality—an experience or belief that no one around a person validates as true (Broussard et al. 2010). People with these experiences try to "make sense" of them in different ways. Psychiatrist James Griffith has argued that resilience and coping stems from a person's ability to find coherence, or make sense of, their experiences. When those experiences defy explanation—such as traumatic events or psychosis—people often feel demoralized (Griffith 2010). They may have difficulty adapting to and coping with such experiences, particularly ones that affect their sense of moral order and their capacity to exercise moral discernment or make choices they perceive to be "good" and that resonate with others' conceptions of the good.

One afternoon in 2004, Maison and I delved further into his psychotic experiences.

"This has been my lovely abode," he told me, "for nine years."

"And a beautiful abode it is," I noted, taking in the scene—a well-kept aquarium, magazine pinups of lovely and scantily clad women, thriving plants.

I propped my tape recorder next to the ashtray, and as the train rumbled through our conversation, Maison struggled to make sense of his psychotic experiences for me.

> MAISON: Where do they come from? Where do those people come from? They aren't over there just like you, but they seemed like they were right over there. I tried to learn and I read. I read about schizophrenia, and I still couldn't learn anything that would tell me about what I was experiencing. It's something that—it seems impossible. It's not imaginable. . . . Can you imagine going through something like that? I mean just imagine the sound and stuff—a boom, boom, boom—and clean pictures of people and weird looking things—well, not really weird, but—how would you feel? You would see and hear, and it would make you paranoid. Until I came to that point where I realized no one else thought this was real. Then it really became hard to deal with. I had to say—go away! Go away! I was so scared of myself. . . . I was so paranoid I was like looking over my shoulder, looking out of the curtains waiting for the police to come get me. Someone knocks on the door and you think—they're coming for me. . . . That was the worst part of my life—the schizophrenic part of my bipolar situation. The schizophrenic part is the worst part. When you get out of that, that is the most terrible part. . . . You can't eat! The food

isn't right. It changes up on you, and you don't want it. No cereal, no grits, no oatmeal when you look at it, it changes up like acid would do. You don't want it.

ME: Right . . .

MAISON: You might go three days, maybe four, drinking soda pop or water, but you can't eat. It's like acid. The food moves around on you. When you're seeing stuff, the pictures out here interfere—the girls dancing and gyrating all to the music and then the food you are seeing as molecules down here. If I look up here I see one thing, and if I look down here it's different.

ME: Right . . .

MAISON: It's exactly like acid like microdot when you start hallucinating. It does the same thing. I took purple haze, and I got the same effect.

ME: Oh, that's kind of cool—

MAISON: No! It was most certainly not cool. I didn't take acid! I didn't choose it! I am not communicating this right if you think it was cool! [Tears begin to fall and he jerks with tics]. To have a schizophrenic attack is the most awful experience. I call it attacks because it—hits you [he claps his hands]. And it goes away, and then you can work on your bipolar. But you can't work on your bipolar if you're having a problem with schizophrenic attacks. That's the thing you take care of first. The lithium and Depakote aren't going to do you any good and you can't give a person a dosage to help until you fix the schizophrenia.[1] Give them more! Take a blood level test, and get to a point where the levels all set,[2] and then they can taper off but until that point until the schizophrenic part is taken care of there's not much you can do with the bipolar, and it's a rough road to travel down.

ME: And then you add in maybe you don't have a home and you don't have any money . . .

MAISON: Ohhhh, don't talk like that. I am getting sick just thinking about it. Exactly. If you're dealing with that type of problem or situation—no food—

ME: Because that's going to make you hallucinate anyway, no food.

MAISON: Correct, that's exactly correct because that's exactly what happens when you haven't eaten in a long time, especially if you don't have the proper coat on, if it's cold out, if you got a problem, and you're out there that's going to make you sick. If you got a problem, that's going to heighten the problem. The only place you can go is the hospital. That's the only refuge. The place a person can kind of heal who really needs help. Find the police or anybody to bring him to the hospital. You seen that person. That person lookin' and lookin', and their eyes are all big like this (makes scary face), like a wild person and he's having a—

ME: Very tough time.

MAISON: He is—I like that. To other people you look like an animal; you look insane. But it's a very tough time.

"The only place you can go"

When Thelma, a peer provider, had a psychotic break in late August 2006 she did what Maison told me most people had to do to manage disquieting psychotic symptoms. She went to the hospital. When I went to visit her, my plastic knife, matches, and candles were confiscated.

"Really? No birthday candles?" I asked. Marigold, another member, and I were there to celebrate Thelma's forty-sixth birthday.

"This morning, Thelma took the plastic-lined pillow case and the cord from the window blinds, tied it around her head, and tried to suffocate herself. So, no."

We made our way down the hall. Thelma sat in the day lounge in a pale, yellow hospital gown.

"This isn't my best color, I know," she mumbled self-consciously. "There is a different color every day. I wish you came on a blue day."

The SyFy channel—a favorite, I often noticed, of people in mental health settings—blared from a small television in the corner. People paced nervously, and the phone bbbrrrring!ed, but no one answered.

A white-capped nurse observed us from her desk. She was not behind glass, but she had a phone next to her. When one young man shouted aggressively at his visitor, a well-appointed elderly woman in a wheelchair, she used her phone to call in two burly orderlies. When the orderlies dragged him out shouting, I felt like I was in a movie.

Marigold and I tried to stay chipper. We presented Thelma with red velvet cake on which Marigold had scrawled her name in yellow letters on white icing. The other patients, all dressed in yellow nightgowns, joined us as we sang "Happy Birthday." Despite their enthusiasm for the cake, they were clearly not well. Everyone's eyes, accentuated by looming pupils, reminded me of black holes.

"That's the expression of too much medication," Marigold commented later.

Thelma's vacuum eyes gazed at me, but not into me. She quivered with rigidity. I knew it was a side effect of the powerful antipsychotic medications the doctors used to stabilize her symptoms.

And then, with no provocation, she began to talk.

"I planned to wade out into the water, slit my wrists, and just float into peace," she said in a monotone. Cake crumbles tumbled from her lips.

Thelma had been in control of her voices for two years when she joined a research study on voice-hearers, she told me. She lost control of her voices, she thought, while trying to figure out how she controlled them.

"It's like when you can't fall asleep because you're thinking about the moment when you fall asleep," she explained.

"Once I tried to pin down how I stopped the voices, I couldn't do it anymore."

When Thelma told the study director about her plan to commit suicide, she called an ambulance. The director promised they would take Thelma to her favorite hospital and help her get her favorite medication from her favorite psychiatrist.

Only one of these promises—her choice of hospital—was kept.

"I don't understand," Thelma droned on. "I don't mind suffering to help others. I wanted to do this research to help others, but I am upset that I lost control again. It makes me want to die. I don't want to leave everyone, but I can't live in the world this way."

The inpatient psychiatric unit had admitted Thelma for attempting self-harm. As soon as Thelma went seventy-two hours without trying to commit suicide (which would take her three weeks to achieve), the unit would release her to outpatient care. She would receive a prescription and a follow-up appointment. About half of the adults treated never show up at that follow-up appointment and so disengage from services (Kreyenbuhl, Nossel, and Dixon 2009).

"This is a big problem," Alex, a middle-aged member who volunteered to talk about recovery to people in psychiatric wards at hospitals, told me. "You don't have the time you used to have. You have to leave before you are ready and stable, and then you get a little stressed, and you fall apart again and end up back in the hospital. It really shakes your sense that you can be okay. They should let you get stable and then toss you out on the streets." Some people I talked to even reported being victimized when they were released in a drugged haze.

Anthropologist Rhodes described this policy as "emptying beds" in order to get people back out into the community—a policy that emerged when the amount of available inpatient psychiatric beds dropped by two-thirds from 1960 to 1994 (Currier 2000; Rhodes 1991). "Emptying beds" was very important because inpatient psychiatric services often were evaluated on the quantity of days patients spent in the hospital (Floersch 2002). Thus, regardless of its utility, anthropologist Rhodes (1991) characterized the psychiatric ward as a place for "movement" rather than a place for rest and recovery. One had to become rational enough not to hurt himself or herself or another person, and then they were released. Many wished they had more options. Some alternatives have been developed—respites where people can go when they are having a psychotic break and avoid the hospital, for example—but they are not widespread.

Thelma did not want to go to the hospital, and she did not want to stay there, either. Unfortunately, for people who are flagrantly psychotic, the hospital is often the only option. It is a place where recovery should begin—and sometimes does when the right balance of medications is found. But it is also a place where someone must go when hopes for recovery are failing, and it was often seen as a return to square one by the members and case managers.

Restoring Rationality

Uncontrollable episodes of "irrationality" are a core clinical feature of psychotic disorders and other forms of madness (Bleuler 1911; Kraepelin 1902). In philosopher John Locke's *Essay on Human Understanding*, he writes: "[Madmen] do not appear to me to have lost the faculty of reasoning; but having joined some ideas very wrongly, they mistake them for truths; and they err as men do that argue right from wrong principles: for by the violence of their imaginations, having taken their fancies for realities, they make right deductions from them" (Locke 1823:109).

In her autobiography, Elyn Saks, who is now a law professor at the University of Southern California, described the experience of irrationality—an experience she had during a major psychotic break in law school. "I don't like the way it feels to walk back to my dorm. And once there, I can't sleep anyway. My head is too full of lemons, and law memos, and mass murders that I will be responsible for. I have to work. I cannot work. I cannot think" (Saks 2007:2).

The *Diagnostic and Statistical Manual* (*DSM-IV*), the widely-known "diagnostic bible" of Western psychiatrists lists several "irrational" mental states under its description of schizophrenia, including distorted thoughts, misinterpretation of perceptions or experiences, beliefs held despite clear contradictory evidence, speech that "slips off track," and providing irrelevant answers to questions (APA 2000:298–299). These states must last at least "a significant portion of time during a one-month period (or for a shorter time if successfully treated) with some signs of the disorder persisting for at least six months (APA 2000:298). The interpersonal ramifications of such behaviors—loss of work, a disruption in education, and family members' sense that one is "gradually slipping away"—all define clinical schizophrenia (APA 2000:302).

In the United States, the reaction to thoughts considered irrational is often one of fear. There is no shortage of stigma surrounding those deemed mentally ill (Gamwell and Tomes 1995; Grob 1994; Shorter 1997). In 2003, 61 percent of US citizens polled thought that people with schizophrenia were likely to be dangerous (PNFCMH 2003). Likewise, Pescosolido and colleagues (2000) found 38 percent of Americans unwilling to be friends with someone having mental health difficulties; 64 percent did not want someone who had schizophrenia as a close coworker.

Despite these fears, if Americans with schizophrenia did not abuse alcohol or drugs, they were no more likely than everyday Americans to commit a violent crime (Monahan et al. 2001). In fact, they were more often victims than perpetrators. In one study, more than one quarter of persons with severe psychiatric disabilities had been victims of a violent crime in the past year, a rate more than eleven times higher than the general population even after controlling for demographic differences (Choe, Teplin, and Abram 2008). Depending on the type of violent crime (rape/sexual assault, robbery, assault, and their subcategories), the chance of becoming a victim ranged from six to twenty-three times greater among persons with schizophrenia than among the general population (Teplin et al. 2005).

Being "irrational" was often neither welcomed by the person having the experience, nor the people around them. For much of American history, people with psychotic disorders have been subject to a variety of treatments intended to eradicate their irrational thought, and (presumably) restore the moral sensibility lost during psychotic experiences. Early psychiatric ideas about how to treat psychosis began with incorrect assumptions, such as that sufferers had an organic neurological flaw (Rush 1786, 1830), were being punished for immoral deeds (Gamwell and Tomes 1995:15; Jimenez 1987:24–25; Tomes 1984), or were the spawn of inevitable intergenerational genetic decay (Porter 2002; Shorter 1997).

Treatments ranged from the holistic "moral therapy" of the Quakers to mechanical contraptions such as Benjamin Rush's "gyrator" on which hyperactive patients were strapped and spun around to stimulate blood circulation (Gamwell and Tomes 1995:32). Over time, these treatments proved ineffective, and dimmed the hopes of restoring rationality for people with persistent psychotic symptoms (Shorter 1997). Then in the 1950s, a compound known as chlorpromazine, a vivid purple dye, dramatically altered the behavior of Parisian patients with schizophrenia.

Historian Caldwell (1978:30) described the scene: "the atmosphere in the disturbed wards of mental hospitals in Paris was transformed; straitjackets, psychohydraulic packs and noise were things of the past! [Parisian psychiatrists] . . . became pioneers in liberating their patients, this time from inner torments, and with a drug: chlorpromazine. It accomplished the pharmacologic revolution of psychiatry."

After the US Food and Drug Administration approved its use in 1955, Smith Kline marketed chlorpromazine to American public hospitals as Thorazine, a front-line treatment for schizophrenia (Shorter 1997). The dramatic results Thorazine had on people prompted one Maryland hospital worker to write: "the wild, screaming patients [became] a thing of the past. Many more patients could go for drives in the country, visit Towson and Baltimore for shopping excursions with or without attendants, go to the theatre, visit art museums, take in athletic contests, and go out with relatives for dinner. Life became more varied and interesting, and improvement was advanced" (Forbush 1971:124–125). Such reports, as the C/S/Xers later pointed out, rarely took into account the perspectives of the patients who had to take these medications and the profound effects this would have on their lives.

After the dramatic "success" of cholorpromazine, psychopharmaceuticals became seen as a potential cure-all for serious emotional distress. Antipsychotic medications were seen as a miracle drug—a tool with which to liberate patients from long-term irrational states. These medications promised to initiate a journey toward moral belonging for people with schizophrenia. Reducing the frequency and intensity of a person's psychotic episodes, historian Grob (1994:231) explained, prompted hope that this kind of therapy might create a calmer and more humane institutional milieu where people could come for a time, recover, and then be released back into the community to lead fulfilling lives.

In the 1990s, prompted by this "pharmacological revolution" in psychiatry, psychiatrist Nancy Andreasen put forth the model of "the broken brain." She asked us to think about schizophrenia as a chemical imbalance in the brain rather than a product of upbringing or social context (Andreasen 1984). This concept has been widely used in western psychiatric rehabilitation clinics to explain to people with schizophrenia why they should take their medications for life.

This "chemical imbalance hypothesis," Kirmayer and Gold have recently argued, is an oversimplified "neo-humoral approach" that glosses over the complexities of neurochemistry for popular consumption, while ignoring the inconvenient fact that despite decades of research, neurotransmitters cannot be correlated with specific functions, behaviors, or disorders (Kirmayer and Gold 2012). Kirmayer and Gold suspected that much of the push to believe that pharmaceuticals can target specific aspects of psychiatric disorder arose from the powerful pharmaceutical companies invested in promoting this concept. Pharmaceutical companies stood to profit from what anthropologist Janis Jenkins aptly called the "pharmaceutical imaginary." In the pharmaceutical imaginary, pharmaceutical drugs bring us closer to our imagined potentials. One could be even better "if only" one had more energy, or could pay better attention, or had an easier time feeling happy, or was always rational (Jenkins 2010).

This was all part of a broader "medical imaginary" that renders people who have a chronic illness "susceptible to hope engendered by the cultural power of the medical imagination" (Good 2001:397). American popular culture is "enamored with the biology of hope," instead of, perhaps, the power of hope that arises from intimate connections between people (Good 2001:407). The hope engendered by the medical imaginary of a "chemical imbalance" originated from good intentions, but it misconstrued the evidence at hand. While this rhetoric may have liberated families from feeling at-fault for a loved one's problems, Jenkins (2010) argued, it did little to solve the existential problems of agency, kinship, and morality that mattered most to people with psychiatric disabilities.

Taking Meds

Western society thus expected people deemed mentally ill to take medications if there was the potential that the medications could help them be more rational. They imagined that this would be a quick fix. Institutions of "care" in the United States are thus often focused on the restoration of people's seeming inability to talk, think, and act in reasoned ways (Desjarlais 1996). In recent years, this has meant a focus on getting people to take their medications—for life. Consumers needed to actively seek the right medication and adhere to prescriptions to suppress psychotic breaks and achieve enough rationality to signal their readiness to make independent decisions (Copeland 1997; Frese et al. 2001; Mueser et al. 2002; Smith 2000; Spaniol et al. 2002). For many people with psychiatric disabilities, people assumed, rationality was within reach if they would just take their medications as prescribed.

By the time the recovery movement came along, practicing medication adherence—consuming antipsychotic medications at a prescribed rate to control the intensity and frequency of psychotic episodes—had become a "best practice" and a primary task of recovery (Anthony 1993; Cohen et al. 1988; DeSisto et al. 1995; Liberman and Kopelowicz 2002; Torgalsboen 2005). Case managers described members who refused to take their medications as noncompliant, unaware of their illness, and stubborn (Kikkert et al. 2006; Lacro et al. 2002; Wright 2012).

The recovery "model" has always been complicated, muddled by competing interests, and unclear. Even so, many advocates from the beginning wanted to allow people to make personal choices about their medications, including refusing medication, taking medications periodically, or taking them in very low, optimized doses. They advocated for a partnership between doctors and patients, a "shared decision-making process" (Deegan and Drake 2006). Federal recovery standards also promoted personal choice, but in more generic terms.

As they developed their model of medication management, Horizons focused on developing members' sense of personal responsibility to consistently manage their own antipsychotic medications as prescribed. They did not, however, actively tap into the knowledge members had cultivated about their own bodies and medications. This was medication adherence as usual, except case managers no longer delivered medications to clients. Members picked up prescriptions on their own. There was little room for members to acquire the medications that worked for them in the doses they desired (as with biker Barry or Thelma when hospitalized), despite their often-extensive knowledge about medications and the effects they had on their bodies. At the same time, medications posed many dilemmas for members, which affected their desire to adhere to treatment regimens that someone else had set for them.

Side Effects

"Why is it that every time I feel better I think it's a good idea to stop taking my medications?" Isaac asked, swooping into the art room.

Bella patted Isaac on the shoulder. "I know what you mean."

"Why would you want to stop taking your medications?" I asked, looking up from my collage, curious to know the peer staff's perspective.

"Well, side effects can make you feel real bad, honey. Real bad. Tired. Confused. Headaches." Henrietta had been taking medications for about 40 years, so she seemed an authority.

"Yeah," Dwayne agreed, "confused like maybe if you are trying to study you shouldn't take it."

"Or if it's making you too fat," Bella chimed in. "I am five feet tall, and used to be 110 pounds, and now I am like 160. Sometimes I want to go off to get my body back. It's bad enough being crazy, but fat and crazy sucks!" People nodded grimly. I heard the fat or crazy dilemma posed often.

"What about you, Isaac?" I asked. Isaac was another peer counselor working for PEP.

"I don't know; it's just that when I feel better I feel like I don't need them anymore. Like if I am recovered, then I don't need to take medications because that's not what normal people do! And, of course, I don't like the side effects. But then, back into the hospital I go."

Several of the members nodded.

Most members took at least three different medications—one antipsychotic medication (e.g., Thorazine, Haldol, or Risperdal), one medication to prevent involuntary movements like Maison's tardive dyskinesia (e.g., Cogentin), and one mood stabilizer (e.g., Depakote or Lithium). Many also used anti-anxiety medications, antidepressants, and sleep aids. Doctors often added drugs as problems arose, but hesitated to take one away.

The members also feared changing a drug "cocktail" that seemed to help. "I am too afraid to go off the ones I have been on," Alex told me, slouching on an office couch in a worn, black leather jacket. We had ducked into one of the offices for an audio-taped interview.

> ALEX: I don't ever want to go back to where I was without them.
> . . . I think the only way to really know who I was before and start over and get it down maybe to a couple of meds is to go in the hospital for a few weeks and just clean my system. Two or three weeks of no meds they say would do it, and then I could start again. It's a shame, but I can't.
> ME: Why not?
> ALEX: Hospital stays are too short these days. It took me three months my first time to get balanced on the meds. It doesn't

happen overnight, you know. My insurance pays for ten days, and then I'm out. It's not enough time to go off carefully and experiment. I would need a lot more time.

A safe, protected space in which to freely adjust one's medication for a few months based on one's personal experiences of side effects was rarely available in the culture of emptying beds prevalent in American hospital psychiatry. And so, despite the promotion of medication adherence and fears about making drastic changes, everyone tinkered with their medications. Members possessed sophisticated knowledge about drug interactions, half-lives, and dosages. When they talked to each other, they strategized ways to cut back or make better use of their medications. Many felt taking medications moved them forward. They remembered a time before medications and after; they typically preferred the after. Even so, they often described challenging side effects, as well.

During one session of the Men's Group with about ten people in attendance,[3] Hank announced, "So let's just get it out on the table—how many of you guys don't want to take medication because then you can't get an erection?"

Everyone looked at me.

"Well that's a major problem for me!" I jested.

Everyone laughed, and the taboo topic became acceptable. They requested that I tell other people about their concerns. They told me that medications limited their ability to have sex or even masturbate. They felt like eunuchs. Many claimed they could not take erectile dysfunction medication due to cardiovascular complications, also potentially aggravated by their antipsychotic medications.

"I am afraid to take a woman out on a date," James sighed. "What woman wants to date someone who can never sleep with them? And then I'd have to tell her why. Forget it!"

Women also claimed to experience sexual dysfunction. They told me that the medications had altered their menstrual cycles. Many had not had a regular menstrual period in years. They worried that the medications were profoundly affecting their fertility, but they had no idea how to address the problem. Their doctors had no advice except to accept the problem as part of their need for medication. Some told me that this made them feel "less than a woman."

More dramatic side effects, such as Maison's tardive dyskinesia, publicly marked people as users of antipsychotic medications. Up to 90 percent of people who used antipsychotic medications for more than three months developed tics and other contractions, and 20 percent developed mild forms of tardive dyskinesia (Casey 1999). Newer medications known as atypical or second generation antipsychotics (SGA) were supposed to help (Jeste et al. 1999; Kane and McGlashan 1995). Extensive research, however, suggested that the new antipsychotics were neither more effective nor better tolerated, although they may cause fewer movement-related side effects (Geddes et al. 2000:1371).

For some, side effects like tardive dyskinesia and weight gain invited stigma (Jenkins et al. 2005). Drugs meant to help people integrate into the community as rational adults also created social distance between those who took medications and those who did not (Estroff 1981:111). Even as treatment began to work, self-stigma against diagnoses and continued medication use remained (Jenkins et al. 2005; Jenkins and Carpenter-Song 2008; Link et al. 1997). These factors, so intricately related to members' abilities to experience intimacy, and so nourish their need for moral agency, only complicated medication adherence.

The Unmedicated

Despite the side effects, with which she had personal experience, Vera believed that life without medication was "Hell." She definitely tried to keep track of her medications.

"The people who don't take their meds, well, they are the worst of the worst," Vera told me, "and God help them, they need us the most." For this reason, Vera allowed people to join the milieu even if they seemed psychotic and were not taking medications, so I had some exposure to people who refused medications for long periods.[4] PEP offered them food, warmth, hygiene, and affection.

They struck me as hauntingly alone, but accompanied by their voices and delusions all the same, which seemed to dominate their thoughts and left little room for socialization. Untreated, flagrant psychosis seemed very disruptive to intimacy and connection to others—far beyond, it seemed to me, the negative side effects of medications that the medicated people who were doing so well described. With this population, Vera advocated "slow engagement" to build trust. Ideally, she said, PEP members would eventually trust someone enough to accept medications.

"Take Ozzie, for instance," Vera told me one afternoon. "I let him in [the center] and he is refusing meds. He thinks it's poison. Okay, but I show him every day when I take my meds. I say, "Okay, I take this poison, and I am doing pretty good." And five, six months later he is asking where I get the meds. Now he's on his way."

"On his way to recovery?"

"On his way to something better than where he was, that's for sure," Vera said, giving me a pointed look.

When Margot first came to the center, she looked exhausted and emaciated. "This woman needs us bad," Vera whispered. Despite Vera's compassion, Margot put me on edge. She seemed to take a perverse joy in shouting obscenities at me. Margot thought my name was Claire and that I had "her money."

When I told her I was just a poor college teacher (imagining this would inspire benevolence), she bellowed, "Well, no wonder the kids are so fucked up these days!" After that, she often sang Pink Floyd's "we don't need no education" when I appeared.

My annoyance frustrated me. The others found it amusing.

"Neely, it's okay," Henrietta teased. "Of course you're stressed. You're the only one who isn't blissed out on meds. You should get some Xanax or Valium!"[5]

One Riverside staff member pointed out to me that people "outside" also had difficulty coping with a neighbor who is shouting from their rooftop at three a.m. or who sends the police next door in a fit of paranoia. How do people like Margot fare "out there" when they cannot control themselves "in here?" Even in the center, people had trouble connecting with Margot because she was so overcome by her voices and delusions. Psychosis powerfully disrupted her ability to connect to others.

Vera refused to turn Margot out. Margot spent the night outside. Vera felt she should at least spend the day inside.

"I wonder why she stays outside?" I asked Lucy one afternoon. Lucy had long, silver braids and four cats at home.

"The shelters won't take you when you're like that," she said. "You can't be that agitated; they'll throw you out. And the hospital would want her to take medications, of course. She doesn't want those, either, so she has to go it alone."

Pierre, a volunteer who ran PEP's kitchen, let Margot work with him. Over a couple of weeks, Pierre developed a system to deal with Margot. He told me that when they were in the kitchen doing dishes and she started shouting, he shouted back at her. He said he had to shout and curse or she did not notice him.

"Margot! Who the hell are you talking to?"

Margot would say a name, and then Pierre would say, "Well, tell so-and-so to shut the fuck up!"

In this way, Margot slowly became quieter for longer periods of time.

After a couple of quieter months, Margot gradually accepted help and affection. At a baby shower the members held for me toward the end of my fieldwork, Margot smiled and offered me a bag full of secondhand baby clothes in a variety of colors. This was an extraordinary gift; Margot had no income and was homeless. Even so, she stayed close to Vera, holding her arm and whispering in her ear. She never shouted anymore. I choked up, remembering how I once dreaded her presence. How intolerant I had been; how little hope I had for her!

"Treat people like a person," Vera would say, "and they will become one." The peers offered Margot a level of intimacy most people did not feel they could offer a psychotic person. Margot used that intimacy to push back against her psychosis and began to respond in kind. She even agreed to sleep in an SRO hotel room, and continued to report to "work" as a volunteer in the kitchen every day. She learned how to be a member in good standing at PEP, and this gave her the tools she needed to start building a moral life—a life that felt good to her and those around her. A life that enabled her to act in a way that gave her access to intimacy and recognition. A life, I would argue, as a moral agent.

The Riff-Raff

Another group of people chose to self-medicate.[6] One morning in Maison's apartment, Rosetta told me that she was so high on crack for so long that she did not even realize she was pregnant, much less giving birth to her fifth child, "until it fell out of my butt." Some members, like Rosetta, found great solace in heroin, marijuana, crack, and alcohol. The members called them "the riff-raff." In addition to the damage to others' recognition of you as a "good" person being a drug addict inflicts in American culture, the consequences of drug use were often extreme for the members.

"Alcohol," Tony told me, "slows you down or deadens you or makes you forget what's happening to you. If you pass out—poof! Sleep. No voices." In the process, Tony told me ruefully, he had also lost most of the details of his sixty-five years on the planet and the respect of his extended family.

"Prostitutes, drug dealers, they just take advantage of mentally ill people," Maison told me. "They can smell us coming from a mile away—oh, there's old Joe. He's talking to those voices again, let's trick him." Anthropologist Luhrmann (2008) has written about how homeless women on the street in the United States find anything preferable to being considered crazy, which marks one as weak in a culture where the weak become everyone's prey. Brodwin (2012) has also written about the awareness of case managers that their clients are preyed upon by criminals and drug dealers.

Was Jonas prey when he lost his flesh? One afternoon, deep in a drug binge, he signed over the title of his car to a crack dealer and gave him his keys in exchange for more crack. When the crack ran out, Jonas found his car on the street and waited for the dealer to return. He did not want his car back; he wanted more crack. The dealer ignored him and tried to drive away. In a fit of despair, Jonas held onto the rear bumper.

"Like a giant rug burn," he told me, showing me his puckered, purple stomach. "Only it was pavement." The skin damage, he told me, extended down his thighs.

"How did you manage to hold on?" I asked him.

"I don't know," he said. "I just really wanted to get high."

These stories abounded. Overdoses. Gangrene. Police brutality after people provoked them in a drug-induced frenzy. Head injuries. Stabbings. And a great deal of prostitution.

Staff allowed the riff-raff to "sleep off their buzz" in the common areas. At times, Riverside staff called the police to escort someone out at closing time. When items turned up missing—ranging from a stereo to paintbrushes to a garish (but prized) painting of Horizons' founder—people immediately blamed the riff-raff.

On a sober day, Frank and I were playing pool when he announced, "80 percent of substance abusers were mentally ill first."

"You think?" I asked him as he sank the eight ball that ended our game.

"I know," Frank insisted. "They were trying to work on their mental illness without even really knowing what was wrong. Depressed? Use some meth or some coke—that will cheer you up! Manic? Use some alcohol. Use some heroin. It's cheaper and easier than health insurance. What's the difference between that and doctor's drugs?"

Around 50 percent of people diagnosed with schizophrenia also had a diagnosis of substance abuse at some point (Bellack and DiClemente 1999; Mueser, Bennett, and Kushner 1995). A dual diagnosis of substance abuse in schizophrenia powerfully complicates recovery (Liberman and Kopelowicz 2002:248). Curious, I started attending the center's daily Dual Diagnosis Recovery Group.

The peer staff leader, Joel, explained the group's philosophy in an interview:

> Many people with schizophrenia and other severe mental illnesses don't fit into Alcoholics Anonymous or Narcotics Anonymous because those groups advocate a substance-free life.[7] Many times they say you shouldn't take any substances, and so people using psychiatric medications feel misunderstood. Some groups even infer that it's weak to take psychiatric medications. If you have schizophrenia and a substance abuse issue, this is not a good situation. The problem with substance users is that they often use the substances to alleviate psychiatric symptoms, so you definitely want them to be taking a medication to help do what their substance of choice was doing for them before.

"Why do people abuse substances instead of taking meds in the first place?" I asked.

"Oh, different reasons. Maybe they didn't know they had the option of meds or maybe they just prefer the street drugs."

"Oh yeah?" I asked.

"Sure," Joel said with a twinkling wink. "I have been clean five years but crack was my drug of choice. Getting high and having fun with friends can certainly seem like a preferable way to deal with mental distress than filling a prescription and seeing a therapist."

"Does it work?" I asked.

Joel looked pensive:

> Yeah, it works, in a way. I mean, what's the other way? Taking a pill that makes people think you're crazy and makes you feel awful? Crack made me part of a group. We would sit in my apartment night after night, talking and soaring. And then I almost died doing it because I just wanted more and more. In search of the ultimate high, you keep thinking—this next hit will be it. Then I lost everything to get it—my job, my savings, my beautiful apartment, and my friends. And then I got help and realized I

had bipolar disorder. That was empowering really. I realized I needed help with that. I needed medication instead of crack.

When Medications Fail

Psychiatric symptoms are episodic—they come and go unpredictably, much like the weather. Medications do not guarantee that a person will maintain a steady condition. Even when people do take their medications, they do not always work as expected.

Despite trying various medications, for example, 10 to 30 percent of patients have little or no change in their psychotic symptoms when they use antipsychotic medications. Up to an additional 30 percent of patients have only partial responses to treatment (APA 2004). Sometimes psychosis "breaks through" to manifest itself regardless of medication usage, particularly when treatment continues over long periods of time (Sheitman and Lieberman 1998). Expecting medications alone to fortify one's rationality over the long-term may not be prudent.

Maison's experiences presented the perfect example.

Two years after we met, I heard Maison's voice reverberating up the stairwell at Horizons' headquarters. We had not seen each other for a few months, and I dashed down the steps in delight. He and Vera conversed loudly in the foyer about the possibility of him working as a peer provider at PEP. I watched from afar, not wanting to disrupt them.

"Okay," he was shouting at her, "well, I could really use some more money!"

"Right." Vera patted him on the arm and walked upstairs.

Before I could signal a hello, Maison pounced on a person entering the foyer from the outside, demanding that they give him more money. The person told Maison he had no more money to give him, but Maison argued on. When another staff member who knew Maison passed by, I touched her arm.

"Hey, who is that person, and why is Maison begging them for more money?"

Maison typically lived comfortably in his Horizons apartment on veterans' benefits and social security. She looked apologetic and whispered, "He'll have to tell you that one, but I will tell you that he is talking to his case manager."

I knew the only case management team in the building we were in was a unit geared toward outreach for people in crisis on the streets. As the case manager moved on into the mobile engagement unit's office, Maison angrily headed for the exit.

"Maison, wait!"

He looked at me dismissively.

"Who was that?" I probed, chewing my nails.

"My case manager." We walked to the black couches in the foyer and took a seat. Then he stood back up.

"I need money!" He exclaimed in agitation.

"I'll spend ten dollars on you, okay?" I said quickly. I felt panicked. My person in recovery, my own "show pony" was in crisis. Besides, I owed him for the sodas, cigarettes, candy, and fried chicken he had shared with me numerous times.

"Do you have a smoke?" He asked.

"Sorry, I quit. . . . How are you?"

"Awful, actually!" Maison plopped back down on the couch like a grumpy teenager.

"First of all, I had to leave my apartment, so I had to switch case managers, and I lost all my stuff, and am staying in a crack hotel again."

"WHAT?" Memories of his happy visitors, aquarium, and plants flashed through my mind. "Maison, you have been living there nine years. How did that happen?"

Maison explained that his morbidly obese neighbor, Roberta, stopped showering. To cover her body odor, she began using a perfume that he felt caused him to hear voices again. He said that he moved out of his apartment to get away from the smell because staff would not intercede. They said she was making her own choices, which was good for her recovery.

"I wasn't trying to hear no more voices because Roberta stinks and has to bathe herself in perfume!" Maison exclaimed. His head jerked with tics. My mind raced. He usually had impeccable grammar.

"Did something precipitate this?" I asked, wondering if this was the whole truth.

"Well," Maison mumbled, "I was in the hospital for a month before."

"What happened?" I asked again, feeling like a broken record. As far as I knew, he had not been to the hospital for eight years.

"My lithium. I got lithium poisoning. Kidney failure. I got real sick, and they said lithium and I are over for good."

Was I dreaming? I thought. This dear man had struggled so profoundly and had come to such a successful place helping others. And now his medications, the one thing he always promised people would be there for them if they just took them regularly were suddenly unavailable to him?

I offered to drive him to his new "crack hotel" from headquarters. I wanted to spend more time with him. I bought him some cigarillos. When he told me he had not eaten in three days, we stopped for lunch. Maison agreed to eat while we caught up, but while I was buying him a meal, he went outside to smoke a cigarillo. I lost sight of him, but twenty minutes later he returned.

"You want to buy this?" He thrust a broken computer printer toward me. "It looks pretty good! I found it in that dumpster behind Arby's."

"Not really. You want this food I bought you? It's getting cold!"

"You got any change from lunch?"

"No, I used a credit card."

"Shit."

Maison went back outside. I could see him through the floor-length windows talking to people on the street and trying to hand them a cell phone. I was afraid to go out there, not sure what he was doing. When he came back in, I demanded to know what was going on.

"I have no money, and I need some beer," he said, his blue eyes filling with tears. "If I can't have Lithium, can I not please have some beer?"

I froze. How was I going to keep him from relapsing? The Maison I knew had been sober for nine years. I remembered his advice—sometimes the hospital was the only place to go. While he erratically nibbled a burger, I offered to take him to his doctor. He agreed.

As we climbed back into my car, I could not believe that driving him to the hospital was my only idea. But he was scaring me. I feared he might hurt himself. He could not come to my apartment due to ethical restrictions on my research. I could take him back to his hotel and stay with him until he calmed down, but he had mentioned that drug dealers were trying to shoot him. What if that was true? With Maison behaving so out of character, I could be in danger. And nighttime would be upon us soon enough, and then what would I do if he got worse? Take him where?

On our drive to the veterans' hospital, Maison smoked two cigarillos at a time—one in each nostril—giggling hysterically, and then crying when it burned. I cranked my window down.

"Neely!" he shouted over the roaring wind, "I am so glad you are taking me away! Here, I know! You tell me a Bible verse, and I will tell you who said it! Then I won't think about beer!"

Once inside the hospital, Maison searched the cafeteria for an "old girlfriend" working as a cashier and stopped by the lab to say hi to his "brother." Everyone looked happy to see him, as though he were an old friend. He insisted we drop by the pharmacy where he loudly demanded more Levitra, "but not Viagra, that shit doesn't work!" It was very embarrassing.

After two hours, we finally made it to his doctor's office on the top floor. Waiting outside next to a fake palm tree, I felt at peace. Surely, this doctor would fix everything.

"I have to calm down or Dr. Ferguson's going to admit me," Maison said nervously. His feet bounced rapidly on the floor.

"Wouldn't that be good?" I asked, thinking how chaotic our day had been.

Maison shot me a look.

Then he smiled. "Let's tell her you're my case manager so you can come in, too."

"Okay," I said, not sure if that was the best plan, but I did want a chance to talk to the doctor.

Once we were in her office, Maison patted me on the arm.

"This is my new case manager, Neely," he said, "and she's so young and sweet, and I know she is worried about me, but really I am fine."

Too embarrassed to say I was not his new case manager, and that I had known him over a year, I fell silent. Maison told her he did not want to stay.

Dr. Ferguson folded her hands in her lap. "He seems a little hypomanic [hyper], but I am not going to make him check in if he doesn't want to. Promise to come back if you feel worse, Maison? Maybe in a few days if you get your things in order?"

Maison beamed.

I could not restrain myself. I told her all about our day, leaving out the part where I was not his case manager, sure she would see the urgency of the situation. She did not.

"I have known Maison for eight years," she said firmly. "We switched his medications recently, and he's just adjusting, that's all. And he can come back and check in if he wants to. It's very difficult to involuntarily admit someone, dear."

My brain whirled. Why would he refuse to be admitted and get his medications fixed? Why was going to the hospital the only help I could conjure up for him?

As soon as we walked out of the front exit, he began to smoke another cigarillo through his nose. All the guys out front roared with laughter. I told him I was leaving.

"Fine," he said. "You were no help anyways."

I fumed all the way home.

But then, I did not see him for a couple of months. In the dead of winter, I received a semi-incoherent voicemail explaining that he was on an inpatient unit south of the city. Despite leaving a 15-minute message begging me to visit, he did not say where he was. The callback number did not work. He did not call again.

No one would tell me where he was, either. You are not a relative, they said. You cannot just find out that kind of information if you are not a relative. But I had no idea how to contact Maison's relatives.

A couple of months later, he showed up at the center. The first time I saw him I was sitting with Azura when he loudly pointed out that she used to work on James Street. For weeks after that encounter, he stumbled in and out of the center, dark as a storm cloud.

Vera warned me to "steer clear" of him, telling me that they were still not getting his medications right, and he was very agitated, not at all himself. But I could not help hovering near the doorway sometimes in the large living room as he played blues standards on the piano and sang. I wanted to be with him, but I did not know how.

The very last time I saw him, he dragged a garbage bag heavy with cigarette butts into the art room and raged at me during a game of Bingo.

"Look at you, a spoiled little white girl who won't share any of her money, her TREASURE. I know she has a treasure! Look at these chips!"

After snatching up a handful of my Bingo chips, Maison stumbled straight out the front doors. I ran up to the kitchen to ask Pierre for a sandwich and some chips. It was not time for lunch, but Pierre understood. Food in hand, I raced back downstairs. Having just finished picking up a fresh batch of cigarette butts, Maison was walking out of the gate.

"Maison?" I shouted, running after him. "Can I at least buy you a pack of cigarettes?" He whirled around to face me and put his nose in the air.

"No. You are not my friend."

"Come on, wouldn't you like to not have to carry that big garbage bag with you for a while? I brought you a sandwich."

He dropped the food in the bag of cigarette butts. I winced.

"Please?"

"Oh, all right," he said, stashing the trash bag behind a hedge.

We walked around the block to the store. He never said a word until I tried to buy him a generic brand of cigarettes.

"Actually, I would like two packs of Marlboro Menthol 100s puh-lease," he told the clerk. Then he took his cigarettes and sauntered away.

Maison lost his position as Horizons' token user or voice of recovery. They no longer paid him to give lectures about taking medications and staying away from alcohol and drugs. When I asked about him, the staff shook their heads and offered the same responses: "maybe he's in a nursing home;" or, "I think he's with another rehabilitation program."

Medications, Moral Agency, and Recovery

Maison's story challenged my belief in recovery. He was doing so well, but as soon as his medicines failed him, his life fell apart. And as soon as things started falling apart, he was expected to go it alone. I realized much later that this was because he had no access to real moral agency inside of or outside of Horizons and, thus, no intimate connections to fall back on despite his nine years of residential treatment there.

In the outside world, Maison was a disabled veteran with a long history of substance abuse living on government benefits and estranged from his family. The only place where he had any credibility was at a Horizons residence, to which he no longer had access. And the staff certainly did not have intimate connections with him, or they never would have taken away his apartment. Inside the world of Horizons, he seemed to have access to moral agency while he was the "show pony," but this was contingent upon good behavior. When he began to have trouble, there was no safety net for him, no web of intimate connections to catch him as he fell. Besides staff, no one outside of Horizons seemed to know he existed, except for me. But what could I have done?

When it comes to Maison, I am full of what ifs—what if I had brought him back to my house? What if I had been more patient? What if there was a place where he could have rested for a few days when he was experiencing symptoms, terribly tempted by alcohol, and had no desire to go to the hospital? What if I had been a better friend rather than expecting a doctor to take care of him? What if I had asked him about the contact information for his children or his ex-wife so that I could have let them know what was going on? What if privacy regulations did not keep me from finding out any of that information so I could help him even after he was not well?

But there is nothing I can do. I check online for news or obituaries. And, I fret—what if he walks right past me, and we never recognize each other? I live a thousand miles away now, but still, I am looking. I long to hear him sing the blues.

STEP TWO: SELF-ADVOCATE

4

> Members don't know how to do
> recovery, and they're used to
> having their hand held.
>
> —*Max, 2005, Horizons
> professional staff member*

> The more I say [about recovery],
> the more cut off I become.
>
> —*Andre, 2006, Horizons
> professional staff member*

A t our first meeting, Vera told me matter-of-factly, "Thanks to PEP, freedom and empowerment at the center are up 40 percent." Vera felt these were important goals. People needed freedom and empowerment, everyone seemed to agree, in order to seek recovery. Recovery advocates promoted "empowerment" as a way to reverse the deleterious effects—increased dependency, for example—of long-term interactions with a paternalistic mental health system (Jacobson and Greenley 2001). For Horizons members, empowerment meant learning how to be autonomous, have courage, and accept responsibility. For many staff, though, empowerment was a slippery concept.

One frigid morning in February 2005, I met up with Shelby. Shelby's clients refused to engage with any kind of service, so Horizons' mobile teams met them on the streets. The widely-praised mobile teams aimed to catch people as they "fell through the cracks." They targeted the homeless—approaching them slowly with a sandwich or a pack of cigarettes, having some casual conversation, and then checking on their mental health needs.

Today we would be meeting with Earl, an African American man in his late forties, at a café in a working-class neighborhood. Shelby carried items Earl requested when they met the week before—new snow boots and two packs of cigarettes.

Earl shuffled in a few minutes late. He was bearded, grizzled, and grey. His eyes lit up when he saw his new boots. When he started to remove his tattered shoes and socks to put them on, Shelby suggested he change his shoes in the bathroom instead.

"We don't want to get kicked out, right buddy?"

As Earl walked toward the bathroom, Shelby leaned across the table. "Let's talk frankly." Her brow rumpled with frustration. "So recovery says that my client has to make his own choices about meds and housing and what he does with his day and how he spends his money all by himself. I don't make him follow any rules . . . and if my member chooses to drown—or even if he just can't swim—then I let him drown?"

I recalled that Melanie, Horizons' Director of Recovery, had recently sent an email to staff members in the agency about their new, "recovery-oriented" policies. The email had stated:

> User choice, user empowerment, and user education about an
> array of life choices have become new fundamental principles . . .
> it is not easy to let go of the privileges and false (but comforting)
> certainties of traditional mental health—for example, that staff
> are the true experts (certainly not users!) on what "is best" for
> someone; that members ought to fit themselves into a schedule and
> system designed to maximize our convenience—not theirs; that
> rigid adherence to rules with strict "consequences" is the only way
> to make a program "safe" and orderly; and so on.

Shelby seemed to have this on her mind as we spoke. "I watch him drown? I cheer him on? Even if he's sixty, and he's been drowning his whole life? Even if he's twenty, and he hasn't ruined his life yet? Recovery says I watch him suffer. Why? I want to buy it, I do. I want it to be right, but I just don't know. I don't know if that's really the best thing for Earl, and I care about him. I don't want to watch Earl drown. I am *paid* to help him."

Staff—Shaken, not Stirred

Shelby was not alone. Many Horizons staff questioned the changes spearheaded by Steve, their new CEO. When Steve first arrived, many people had been moved around the agency—promoted, demoted, and even fired. Steve told me that he purposely "shook up the staff" to break down the established order. He also created a new Chief of Clinical Operations and a senior administrative position (now Melanie's) for a peer Director of Recovery. For an organization that had been under the same CEO for several decades, these were substantial changes. When I said as much during an early conversation, he assured me that all evidence-based organizational culture change takes ten to twelve years. At this point, we were at the beginning of the third year of the change process.

As I began to talk to people, I found that staff seemed concerned. "I am almost reluctant to use the word recovery because it's so emotionally laden," Jacob, Riverside's Program Director told me. "Hook them [staff] up to the recovery machine, and there's a spike in blood pressure." He winced and clenched his fists over his heart, making it clear that the spike was painful. "Recovery has been cast in a punitive light like we need to divorce the past from what we do now. Well, what did we do wrong, and what do we do now? It's not just the word recovery, but how it plays out. The staff feel an extreme self-consciousness and angst."

Around the same time, Horizons' Recovery Steering Committee released a new organizational "mission statement" promising to make all of Horizons' programs exemplars of recovery, where messages of hope, choice, and wellness could be conveyed to staff and members. A "key concepts of recovery" pamphlet distributed to staff also highlighted "personal autonomy," "voice," "active participation" and "partnerships."

At one meeting, Barb showed an article to the steering committee that suggested focus groups were helpful *before* any organizational changes were made. "Why not retroactively check in?" she asked, smiling at me. The Recovery Steering Committee asked the Research Department to conduct focus groups. The Research Department then asked me to conduct the four anonymous, randomized focus groups (I did three). They wanted me to accentuate my position as an "outsider," which would keep all of the data confidential since I would not know anyone, and people might speak more freely with me. While I did know some people at Horizons at this point, I definitely did not know most of the staff at the one hundred programs that Horizons supervised, and many were drawn from programs I had not visited. I did not personally know any of the focus group participants, although I did recognize two of them as leaders in the organization. The Research Department anticipated a glowing article about staff satisfaction with a complicated change process that would put Horizons on the map as a leader and indicate ways forward. Staff were randomly sampled from across the agency so that the focus group findings would be more generalizable to the whole agency. The Research Department wanted to publish the findings in a good journal.

Instead, the focus groups were rather negative in content. Many staff shared their discontent. They did so hesitantly, and only after much reassurance that they would remain anonymous. What follows is derived from detailed notes that I took during the focus groups, which the Research Department let me keep.

Bruce, a man who I later found out had held a broad range of positions at Horizons over decades, spoke his mind at one focus group. "A lot of people wrestled with—why are we doing recovery for members but treating staff like they're expendable? The way recovery was rolled out as an agency initiative felt very paternalistic toward staff, and staff picked up on that."

A female case manager agreed with him. "Case managers are at ground zero of all these ideas and rules, and it's not easy given what they have to work with.[1] You want to empower people, but it only makes the members against us feeling worse. Recovery aggravated this and made it sound like staff was the enemy blocking the route to a better life. This message was put out there by administrators even though we case managers are really trying to help people."

Bruce continued to challenge the recovery philosophy during a later interview:

> So recovery wants me to give Bob his whole disability check at the beginning of the month so he can choose what he wants to do with it rather than me doling it out so he can eat and have a shelter. And I know full well he is going to use it in those first few days to rent a hotel and smoke crack and get a prostitute because if he has enough money to have a good time he will pursue one. And I know the rest of the month he will be broke, sick and tired, and homeless, and I will be almost powerless to help him with no money. Oh, yeah, and I am not supposed to help because he has to take personal responsibility for his choices. And that's recovery?

Bruce looked down at his hands and shook his head:

> Don't you think if poor life circumstances were going to inspire Bob to change they already would have? No, he's going to overdose. Or get HIV. Or get really addicted and steal to get more and then go back to jail. Or get beaten or shot or stabbed by a prostitute for those new boots. Or fall down in the snow and freeze to death. And I have to call his family and tell them I was trying to help him recover but he's dead or—worse—sicker than when I opened his case.

Seasoned case managers like Bruce, I noted, often shared the wizened look of their clients. Overworked and underpaid, they took up their clients' yokes when their clients set them down. They fought for people's survival when people did not care to survive. They navigated the labyrinthine circuit of institutional care daily. They carried the burden of guilt when a user experienced rehospitalization, and they accepted the agony of having clients who committed suicide, died prematurely, or disappeared. Every day they needed to be reasonable, compassionate, supportive, and hopeful.[2] They worried that their clients would languish without direction. They seemed to almost be pleading me to tell them—how does one *provide* recovery? But they also seemed to have little faith that recovery was even possible for the members.

Bruce looked at me thoughtfully. "You seem really optimistic, and I don't want to squelch that. We're going to try, but consider the possibility that we might fail—just like the members. Is that okay, if staff fail, too? You might really burn out staff this time. You might take the occasional reward of six months of stability for our members away from us. Then what are we there for? Who will give us the hope to be hopeful?"

Other, often younger (and perhaps more optimistic and less burnt-out) staff seemed to appreciate recovery policies, which they felt added a new dimension to their interactions with members. Max and I chatted as we drove around one morning searching the nooks and crannies of downtown skyscrapers for one of his homeless clients. Then we settled on floor cushions in his office to chat with another staff member.

"It's harder for staff to make changes and let people suffer life consequences," Max told me.

"It's not so much that staff know better," Jane said. "We learned from experience and the members need to learn, too. Like going away to college."

"Yeah," Max said. "Let them learn. Some people may need hands-on, but a lot can manage more than we think."

"We all do it every day and live with the consequences," Jane said. "Case managers just have to figure out where the gap is for the member between what is okay—what the person is able to do and what they aren't."

But really, this was the hardest part. Figuring out what members could and could not do was difficult when seasoned members possessed little sense of their own capabilities, older staff claimed.

"Members don't know how to do recovery, and they're used to having their hand held," one case manager told me during another focus group.

"Right!" another case manager said. "Members are used to us being more paternalistic, and now they think we're hanging them out to dry," he said. "They were not at the trainings. They think recovery is some substance abuse thing. We need more time and staff to teach them what's going on."

"It's scary for some members," another person agreed. "For the past twenty years, we have fostered dependence, and now it's scary for them to do it by themselves. We have to teach them how to do it. Will the members shave before job interviews if I don't remind them? Will the members spend their whole check on cigarettes instead of housing and food?"

Another added: "When I started a year ago, senior staff was very paternal and protective, but now even the old birds in the nest are moving toward independent living! I see more hospitalizations with my clients, which might be one problem with the model. Some members can't handle the stress of change and choice."

Even though Horizons' recovery philosophy stated those members' failures were a necessary and natural part of the journey of recovery, signs of failure made case managers wonder if recovery was really abandonment. Mabel spoke of her reservations as we drove to drop psychiatric medications off to a member. We both knew that the recovery model sought to eradicate medication drop-offs, but this annoyed Mabel.

"Recovery needs to be more specific," she groaned. "Right now it seems like a yellow brick road leading in every direction! Some people would sit in a chair all day and call it recovery if they weren't told what to do! Recovery isn't sleeping all day! Firmness and direction are a necessity! An agency needs to be firm and directive."

Mabel really hated the new rules that allowed people to sleep in the TV rooms and did not require them to attend therapeutic groups if they did not want to do so:

> We need to tell people they would benefit from a group. . . . The pendulum is swinging between firm structure and soft fuzziness, and I think we should swing back more in the other direction. These people are ill and giving them a soft option isn't really what they need. Recovery from a car accident isn't all fuzzy. We don't want recovery to be only soft and mushy. It could be recovery from a cold, and you'd still need a doctor! These people need firmness— they wouldn't be here if they didn't need us.

At times, the Recovery Steering Committee heard about strong rejections of recovery initiatives across the agency. Andre was a key informant on this issue for the committee. He was hired to help lead the frontline initiative at one program as a recovery-oriented case manager. At one meeting in 2005 that I attended, Andre, a program director named Lee, a senior administrator named Barb, and a Horizons member/peer trainer named Lynn had this telling conversation.

> ANDRE: The more I say [about recovery], the more cut off I become.
> LEE: Recovery requires a shift in the self-concept of the worker. They have a messiah/ savior complex. "Oh, I am healthy, and you're not, and I know what your goals should be."
> BARB: Some people are unhappy people. . . . They give immature feedback.
> LYNN: Even as trainers we run into that and don't want to go [do the training] because you get beat up every time you do it!
> BARB: Some people should have been fired a long time ago. They resist anything new. . . . We need our best people to turn the ship. . . . Andre, we'll help you find another job at Horizons. . . . The shit hits the fan with recovery—and Andre, you landed in the fan.

LYNN: Well, the good news is you landed on the blade. And my two cents as a member—people who are willing to stick their necks out make a real difference in people's lives, and it's so important.

A month later, I made an entry in my field notes: "[Andre] is still whiny and is taken less seriously now. He needs to be more constructive in his criticisms—people [on the committee] are just nodding at this point—and he is very guarded about his capabilities/what he can and cannot do for the recovery efforts at Horizons."

Barb never found Andre a new position at Horizons. He resigned a few months after I made this note. He claimed there was not enough organizational support for change. Administrators said they were "sorry to see him give up," and then business continued as usual. The CEO, Barb reminded us, had said that organizational changes would take ten years.

Despite the obstacles, some Horizons staff became cautiously optimistic, including Riverside's Program Director, Jacob. Six months after his initial comments about recovery as a "machine" to which staff would not want to be hooked up, he offered an alternative perspective. "The recovery philosophy makes us focus on hope instead of maintenance, and empowerment instead of service needs," he proclaimed. "To me, it's like taking me back to Horizons when it started where there was more camaraderie with members, and the relationship was not so confrontational. We're not asking, 'what am I going to do?' but 'how can I help you do what you need to do?' We are encouraging people to be more independent—that's a good thing." Jacob found it reassuring, he told me, that Horizons was "going back to go forward," which he had come to see as a return to the past rather than a negation of previous efforts.

Other Horizons case managers continued to suggest that they felt caught in a Catch-22. They were supposed to let members try, fail, and learn to take responsibility for their choices, but also help them make "good choices" that posed no threat to themselves or others. Case managers perceived this as a thin, fuzzy, and arbitrary line between neglect and empowerment. Recovery advocates would say they were being too paternalistic.

"Good" Choices

People with psychiatric disabilities were routinely refused the opportunity to make their own choices (Estroff 2004; McCubbin 2001; Stefan 2002). Even though psychosocial rehabilitation programs allegedly encouraged user choice and partnership with mental health professionals (for example, supported housing [Carling 1995], the clubhouse model [Beard, Propst, and Malamud 1982] and case management programs [Pyke, Lancaster, and Pritchard 1997; Rapp 1998]), many argue that these models engendered paternalistic relationships. Case managers often thought clients lacked awareness of their illnesses, were vulnerable, and could not act in their own self-interest (Angell, Mahoney, and Martinez 2006). Social workers aimed to compensate for a client's presumed lack of competency, even though they often did not themselves have the power or knowledge to make a difference (Brodwin 2012; Wright 2012).

Floersch's (2002) ethnographic work beautifully illustrated the gradual (and often well-intentioned) process through which a case manager using a "strengths-based" model came to be in control of most aspects of their client's lives despite the model's intention of building the client's strengths. First, case managers created a "working alliance" or "therapeutic alliance" between themselves and their clients (Walsh 2000). They then used their relationship to develop the client's treatment plans based on their "strengths," but these plans nearly always focused on medication management, money management, and behaving properly in public—or "meds, money, and manners" (Angell 2006; Christensen 1997; Davis 2002; Floersch 2002; Rowe et al. 2001). Over time, case managers made many decisions for their clients.

The ability to make one's own choices, I would argue, is a fundamental precondition for moral agency, at least in western countries (Brock 1993; Buchannan 2008; Buunk and Nauta 2000; Crisp and Hooker 2000; Dworkin 1988). "Good," healthy citizens have the right to pursue their own, "enlightened" self-interests as moral agents. Enlightened self-interest was not only morally good in the United States, but also thought necessary for the well-being of all.[3] When acting on one's own behalf in an enlightened way, moral citizens contributed—even if inadvertently—to the greater good (Smith 1904 [1776]). Being systematically denied the ability to make choices by institutional policies was demoralizing for Horizons members.

I witnessed members' lack of choices at many of the Horizons programs I visited. Staff controlled access to landlords and public housing programs and decided where members lived and with whom. They controlled access to the members' bank accounts as their "payee," and decided what members could afford to buy. Good behaviors, if the member was lucky, might be rewarded with a little extra spending money. Staff also planned and ran most program activities at the center, and many suggested activities that were not "billable" were not worth pursuing. Staff also dictated when, where, and how often members should take their medications. I watched staff deliver medications to clients' homes to watch them swallow—with water because clients could spit their pills into soda or milk.

Staff also had to decide whether or not erratic behavior required members to be hospitalized, sometimes against their will. During one visit to a Horizons program, I was informally visiting with clients in a living area, chatting with them about their everyday lives. One of them, Lucinda, was very excited because it was her birthday. She said she was not allowed to have cake because (for whatever reason, there may have been a good one) the staff said she could not have one. As she said this, though, she pointed to a picture of a birthday cake on the bulletin board, and said—"but I could have some of that cake!" She then jumped up, ran to the wall, and licked it eagerly a few times. A frazzled-looking case manager entered just as she did so. Later, as I was talking to the staff behind a bullet-proof glass window in the staff room, the case manager called for an ambulance. Lucinda was hospitalized for licking the wall. The case manager said it showed that she was not thinking rationally enough to be living independently. I tried to explain about the birthday cake and Lucinda's birthday, but she looked annoyed and told me that it did not matter.

Case managers also often resorted to what anthropologist Brodwin (2008:139) called "informal practices of surveillance," such as searching a client's trash for beer cans or demanding information about drug use, prostitution, and drinking. Staff asked who the members had visited, what they ate, and where they spent their days. To the average American, this seemingly Orwellian "Big Brother is watching" invasion of an adult's privacy might seem appalling. Brodwin (2008:139) and others have argued that many case managers felt confused by their coercive relationship with users (Angell 2006; Angell and Mahoney 2007; Davis 2002). They wanted to grant their clients more autonomy, but—as with the staff I met at Horizons—abandoning or neglecting their clients concerned them (Brodwin 2008).

Even so, Horizons' administrators claimed to be on a mission to promote member choice and empowerment. In one all-agency memo, Melanie wrote:

> The user's number one complaint is boredom. My mission is to speak on behalf of the notion that life is rich, interesting, and full of possibilities, so get out there and experience your self as a person who is on a great adventure. There are lots of detours and catastrophes but that is part of the journey—it's grist to the mill— take risks, make mistakes, learn, and grow. Come in and be alive with your best game on.

The Dignity of Risk

Like Vera and Melanie, national recovery advocates promoted empowerment and choice as keys to recovery. Activist Patricia Deegan (1996) wrote "[we] are not objects to be acted upon. We are fully human subjects who can act and in acting, change our situation. . . . We can become self-determining."

At the Alternatives 2006 conference, another peer provider and recovery activist Amy Jones explained her position:

You've been in the system a long time and you see all the important decisions are made by them [mental health professionals], so you think—why try? Because you're compliant. They want you to be compliant and reinforce it by giving their approval when you are. They say—that's a great choice! Who do you say things like that to? Kids. I don't care if you think it's a great choice or not. Compliance stops critical thinking. We are forgetting to ask why. Why is it a great choice? What goes into that decision-making? We've been compliant too long. We need to start asking questions about decisions and making our own. Sometimes we won't make a good decision. Then we'll learn. We'll learn to weigh the costs and benefits so that we're not afraid to deal with reality. The key isn't to be rewarded. Why do we teach consumers that the only way to get what you want is to wait for someone to give it to you?

Recovery advocates like Jones wanted providers to help clients practice self-determination rather than coercing them (Anthony 2000:7; Farkas et al. 2005). They argued that users needed opportunities to acquire skills to manage their own lives (DHHS 2003b:1–3).

To help them accomplish this, psychiatrist Mark Ragins (2002) wrote that recovery-oriented staff should: "cease all caretaking and protective practices." Psychologist Larry Davidson (2009:167) thought that case managers still needed to believe in their clients when clients could not believe in themselves. Case managers, advocates believed, should also have genuine hope that users could heal (Crowley 1996; Kruger 2000; Mead and Copeland 2000; Pierce 2004). Advocates also wanted case managers to let consumers make their own choices—even bad ones (Deegan 1996:5; Mead and Hilton 2003; Schiff 2004; Solomon and Draine 2001). Consumers, advocates claimed, deserved the "dignity of risk"—the right to make bad decisions and fail like every other adult (Deegan 2003; Hopper 2007a; Mead and Copeland 2000). I would agree that taking risks was one of the few ways members could develop the capacity to effectively practice moral agency. If a person is going to learn to act in a way that resonates with others, there has to be some room for practice, failure, and second chances.

Peer provider Amy Jones compared the dignity of risk to getting a speeding ticket. "We learn from these experiences of failure," she said, "and know what not to do again." From this process, advocates argued, people learned to accept their own limitations and develop a sense of their own potential (Deegan 1988:14–15). Consumers, Ragins (2002) advised, needed to embrace relationships with staff that allowed them more self-responsibility. This meant that users should also give positive feedback to staff who gave them more control over their own lives rather than blaming them if things went wrong. They needed to recognize staff that let them make choices and fail as good and valuable people. Developing "an active and effective sense of self as a social agent," advocates hoped, would keep consumers from learning to be helpless (Sells, Stayner, and Davidson 2004:88). Staff, I might add, also needed to develop a stronger sense of self as a moral agent to combat the demoralizing obstacles they face working at the front lines of community psychiatry—high futility, poor resources, and also being on the "lowest rung" of the professional ladder in terms of salary and power (Brodwin 2012).

By learning to make their own choices again, advocates hoped people in recovery would regain access to their "inalienable rights." In his keynote address, Alternatives Conference speaker Ed Knight defined these "inalienable rights." Many of them took the form of resources that would improve one's ability to become a moral agent, like respect, food, shelter, medical care free of cruel and unusual punishment, the capacity to not give in if you don't want to, not to have your information shared, and the right to refuse treatment.

Horizons members had not been taught to understand the dignity of risk as part of recovery. One afternoon, Barnie, the president of the All Agency Members' Council, sat down with me to enjoy our free sandwiches after a meeting. During this time, he told me:

> I have a rent payee. I suck at money. And I've been told that this
> is a problem with recovery. A hindrance. I have bad credit, and no
> checking account, and so I have a rent payee. Part of my recovery is
> realizing that I have a problem with money and need a rent payee.

People need to stop telling me this is a problem, people! If it's your choice, then it's recovery, right? And if I do have a relapse, then someone knows to pay my rent, so I won't get evicted and lose all my stuff! Geez!

Recalling how quickly I had seen possessions outright disappear off a city street during an eviction helped me appreciate Barnie's point. Many members lost belongings during evictions. However, Barnie's continued dependence on their help to pay his rent contributed to staff's doubts that he would ever be able to recover.

Troublemakers

He was, in turn, not afforded much dignity. One senior administrator told me that the staff regarded him as "a joke." They all stopped listening, this person told me, when Barnie started talking because he went on and on about irrelevant things, and he rarely delivered what he promised. No one bothered to tell Barnie, though, which may have helped him practice being a better speaker so that he could accrue some moral agency in that setting.

The staff had no idea why he had been elected as the president of the Member's Council, but I did. Barnie was fearless, articulate, and a good advocate, even if Melanie frequently shut him down for going "off the agenda." At one point, the administration promised to give the next elected Members' Council president a seat on Horizons' Board of Directors. This offer was meant to excite members and entice someone else to run.

They wanted someone more "recovered" to oust Barnie (the sitting president), a senior administrator told me. But if he remained as president? I asked.

"Are you kidding me? Barnie will never be given that role. Can you imagine?" The Board might have been surprised, it was true, to hear someone advocating "off the agenda," but it was probably just what Horizons needed.

Many members participated in the election and Barnie was re-elected. After his re-election, the administration appointed a peer attorney to the Board instead. Barnie's tireless advocacy, clearly respected by the members, made no difference except to invite a dismissal by senior staff.

Why would members want to advocate for themselves if nothing changed and they lost credibility? Barnie was not advocating for complete independence. He was, however, making tentative steps in advocating for his fellow members, which could have inspired recognition rather than ridicule.

This exchange between Melanie, Barb, two members—Ella and Lynn—and myself at a Recovery Steering Committee meeting illuminated more reasons why members might be reluctant to self-advocate.

> MELANIE: So Mortimer [a member] called and was discouraged. I called their supervisor and we talked and met with the member. The staff member resented that this wasn't her primary client, and she was having to deal with a complaint the member made. "Really, Mortimer," she asked, "don't you think you could do this yourself?"
>
> BARB: That sounds empowering.
>
> ME: Well, wait—was her tone demeaning like you just made it sound?
>
> MELANIE: Demeaning? That staff member treated Mortimer as if he were retarded! It was *not* empowering.
>
> BARB: Did they treat you like that, too?
>
> MELANIE: No, but if I hadn't been there, I don't think anything would have happened at all! He had already tried to talk to his case manager and two program directors.
>
> ELLA: And members are afraid to speak up. You get labeled a troublemaker. You follow your little handbook guidelines, and you get ignored. And then you're afraid of losing your housing. I hear that all the time—well, if you don't like it, then you can live somewhere else. That's not empowering. It's the opposite.
>
> LYNN: I agree with Ella. I get threatened and hear people get threatened with housing all the time.

Barb: Well, there are pockets of poison in the organization—
people who just don't get recovery. We need to get rid of those
staff, and we will, but it's going to take time.

Ella: That doesn't make me feel any better about my housing,
honestly. Until Horizons can guarantee that members speaking
up for themselves won't just be seen as just talking back, a lot of
people are going to stay quiet.

Ella was a strong-willed woman who rarely hesitated to speak
her mind. She ran for Members' Council President, and came in
second. But even she recognized that "staying quiet" rather than
"talking back" made good, common sense. The potential backlash
of self-advocacy was not worthwhile, she said. Members earned
preferential treatment in housing, employment options, and volunteer opportunities with good, compliant behavior. Such behavior also promised a minimal but satisfying sense of intimacy
with staff.

This meant that the kind of moral agency members had to develop
in the center to secure a little intimacy with the staff—dependence,
compliance, staying quiet—did not mesh with what was being
promoted by the organizational philosophy—independence, self-
advocacy, and personal choice. And it seemed that when the members
changed their activities as moral agents to match that of recovery, they
were no longer recognized as "good" people by the staff.

In addition, certain perks that members received—funds
to have a jazz brunch, a new pair of shoes, or a cup of coffee at
Starbuck's were not always "billable." If someone could not be
billed for a service members received, then these perks became a
favor. Recovery-oriented self-advocacy, members of both PEP and
Riverside worried, might lead to fewer favors if staff became irri-
tated with them. Complicity cultivated tranquility and stability in
this institution's culture. Desjarlais (1996:886) described similar efforts of tactical agency among the homeless, "mentally ill" shelter
residents with whom he worked, who often used "various tricks
and ruses and other calculated actions" when the chance arose to

accomplish what they wanted in a system in which they had little, if any, power. Few members showed any active interest in advocacy work. Those who did, like Barnie, faced the possibility of ridicule and lost the little moral agency they had in these settings.

One afternoon, Ella spoke up in a Member's Council meeting that was starting to run over time. She had been finding her voice in the past few months, I had noticed, and was doing less "staying quiet" and more advocating. Perhaps she was a bit assertive, her metaphor to describe tensions between staff and members a little crass (something about how members should not have to "spread their legs" to please staff), but her comments were relevant. But to my surprise, Melanie, who directed the meetings, sharply cut her off. She said, "Ella! That is not appropriate!" No one said anything else, and the meeting ended there.

Later, Ella told me that she was stunned. She considered Melanie a friend and peer, so how could Melanie dare shame her by telling her that her ideas were "not appropriate"—a frequent form of staff dismissal that the members found to be infantilizing. Melanie defended herself, telling me that people who had been sexually abused could have negative memories that such comments could "trigger."

After that, Ella remained silent, and the AAMC meetings became much less exciting. When people were afraid to lose the tiny bit of moral agency they had at Horizons by self-advocating, they hesitated to participate. Instead, the meetings became a distribution point for organization initiatives—a place where staff could pass out stacks of fliers for the representatives to take back to their programs and a place for representatives to get a free lunch and a $25 voucher, but not much more. Some staff pointed to this as evidence that the members were just in it for themselves, and not for the agency's betterment.

In another move to promote self-advocacy, each year Horizons bussed 300 members to the state capitol. Once there, the members visited their representatives, handed out information packets, and participated in a rally on the capitol steps. Photos from this event frequently appeared in Horizons' publications.

Prior to the rally in 2006, at an AAMC meeting, Wade respectfully asked for more information about recovery. He said that he looked forward to participating, but needed more information. Barnie; Mona, a state-level peer advocate; Aaron, the peer attorney recently appointed to Horizons' Board of Directors; and Melanie were all in attendance.

WADE: The Horizons theme for the rally this year is Recovery Rocks. We need to educate legislators about what this means. Does it mean drugs and alcohol recovery?

MELANIE: No, it does not.

WADE: Maybe Mona can explain it? What is the legislative agenda?

MONA: There are a number of things we are working on. The day of the rally will be shaped by legislation up to that point. Right now, there are twenty-five pieces of legislation on the table.

MELANIE: We'll spell it all out as we get closer. Basically, traditional treatment was based on a medical model, but socially responsible mental health services look more like refugee services than a mental health system.

WADE: What does that mean?

MELANIE: No more—sorry, but you're homeless. No more ambulances and restraints, but a lot of resources and listening and meeting people where they're at. We show up at jail or at the library and help young women pay for a room at our expense—over and above medical necessity. We reach out to connect people back to support and help. The medical model says—oh, we'll fit you in when we can. Here's some pills. Go away.

AARON: Nothing about us without us. We decide what getting better means and what it is.

WADE: That makes sense, but I am looking at the big picture. There are lots of people in the mental health system who are unable to decide. How do we put a system in place to meet the needs of individuals?

MONA: That's a good question, but right now I need help with the rally.

WADE: But what's our agenda for the rally?

MONA: We aren't capable of coming up with solutions. The point of the rally is to educate legislators about recovery so they know what's possible, and to ask legislators to take appropriate action.

BARNIE: But I agree with Wade! We need to say what recovery is and what to do about it.

MELANIE: Let's work on that more specifically in March. You need to put your body on the line for now. Show up, bring your families, friends—the more people there are, the more press coverage. We need to show them we can organize.

BARNIE: We do that every year. I thought this year was going to be different.

WADE: We're only going to be there for one day, and we need to understand what the recovery model is!

AARON: This is a big process. We can't just tell you in a half hour.

WADE: Last year, I had the ear of my senator, and I didn't know what I was talking about. I was embarrassed.

AARON: We'll do it better this year. Thanks for reminding us.

WADE: Well, as soon as I figure out what recovery is, I will feel better.

AARON: [winking at Wade] I will, too.

On the way to the rally, Horizons staff handed out blue rain slickers and signs with "Recovery Rocks" scrawled in big letters. They also gave us folders with packets of information on "our position" on several mental health-related issues. There was a pretyped letter we could sign and put in an envelope with our senator's name on it also outlining "our position" in bullet points. On the bus, the members around me commented that they did not even understand the comments, but it was worth the free bus ride out of the city. When Wade commented that we were just delivering Horizons propaganda, some members laughed.

After clearing a very long security line at the state capitol building, eight of us somewhat cheerfully plunged through the door of our own senator's office. He was not in. His secretary looked wide-eyed as Moe, a rather large, bearded man with glasses, passed her a large stack of envelopes with our letters in them, as well as the position document prepared by Horizons' administrators.

Wade and I were from different zip codes, so we did not go in together. On the bus ride home from the rally, though, I asked Wade if he felt like he accomplished more this year.

"Maybe a little more," he said hesitantly. "I didn't actually see a senator this year, so it wasn't as big of a deal . . . but I still felt like people were telling me what to say without telling me what it meant. I still want to know more about recovery."

These scenes all depict ways that members who did join meetings and events for member self-advocacy were often not taken seriously. The same "token" users typically attended organizational events, like Maison (for a time), Lynn, and Ella, which limited significant provocations for change (McLean 2000). When newcomers like Wade tried to provoke discussions on relevant issues, senior staff (always in attendance to "guide" meetings) accused them of going "off the agenda." "We need to move on" emerged as the standard phrase to curtail members' earnest inquiries.

To encourage attendance, participating members received a free lunch and monetary reimbursement for their time. But members often had to repeatedly request the promised check, always distributed well after participation was over (typically $25, six to twelve weeks later). The delay signaled a fundamental disrespect for members' time. Staff did not receive their paychecks six to twelve weeks after the fact. And members' repeated inquiries about when they could expect reimbursement led staff to grumble: "members do not care about recovery; they just care about getting a free meal and twenty-five dollars for cigarettes." Again, compliance and staying quiet was the way to garner moral agency in such a setting rather than self-advocacy causing the recovery approach to be ineffective for members.

"Take back what is ours"

Horizons' Recovery Steering Committee felt that they had tried to disseminate some information about recovery outside of the administrative meetings. They hosted the Members' Expo where Vera gave her rousing speech in 2004. The Education Sub-Committee meticulously rescripted official organizational statements like the mission statement, which appeared in a glossy new members' manual featuring photos and bios of members who had not all given permission to be featured (as one of those featured angrily pointed out to me).

The Recovery Steering Committee also printed 4,000 dual-sided, wallet-sized, laminated "recovery cards" with one side for staff and one for members—a symbolic reminder, to the anthropologist, of the strength of the entrenched dichotomy even in targeted efforts to break it down. The "staff" side used plain, directive English: "communicate a belief that a person can and will recover;" or "do not judge, dismiss, or advise." The "member side" was more vague. Answers to a question at the top, "what is recovery?" included: "overcoming internalized stigma"; "reclaiming and strengthening roles beyond being a user in the mental health system"; and "actively self-managing one's life and wellness." These were not clear, directive statements. Some members felt that they needed a dictionary to understand them, they told me. No one found them particularly useful. Thousands of the cards remained undistributed, "in a box in a closet somewhere" six years later, according to one administrator.

There were also virtually no resources for members to connect and organize social change. My research occurred when only a few people had a cell phone (I only had one the last few months of fieldwork), and most did not have email accounts. Members rarely (if ever) called each other on the phone, which cost thirty-five cents. Messages left with staff at residences were not necessarily passed along quickly or fully. Program bulletin boards required someone to create, print, and post a flier. Members typically lacked the resources—paper, markers, or word processors—to try. Bulletin boards mostly displayed institutional policies such as directions in case of an emergency, and few people bothered to look at them regularly. Few Horizons programs had computers or Internet access. Most members did not have an email account (and when I tried to set one up for them, it seemed very hard to explain because most had almost no computer literacy). And the twenty or so members who regularly attended the Members' Council meetings to bring informational fliers back to their programs about agency initiatives did not adequately represent the one hundred programs operating within Horizons.

Ella, who did not attend PEP because she worked full time and it was pretty far from her residence, imagined everything was different there, where the peers ran the show. "So much of recovery is a window dressing—it looks like something is happening and the people in power point to it as evidence that something is happening, but it's a set," she said at one Recovery Steering Committee. "PEP is real. It's really changing things—expected and unexpected. It's really a true, ground-up initiative that is all user-driven. We are hoping to change the system with a ripple effect." However, since Ella was never a member of PEP, she rarely glimpsed what happened backstage.

Backstage, Vera busily orchestrated the show. Noticing members' reluctance to self-advocate, Vera hoped that making autonomous choices as a group would strengthen members' confidence. By teaching members to "take back what is ours" in the mental health system, Vera believed, members would take back control of their own lives. At least, this is how recovery began to grow in her own life.

Over a decade ago, Vera told me, she was a "compliant mental patient" at a suburban community mental health center when she heard a city worker tell a fellow patient, "Get out of my way, you crazy bitch." He wanted to set up his ladder to change a light bulb, and she was in the way. After setting up the ladder, he went back outside to obtain a new light bulb from his truck. While he was gone, Vera—who claimed that at this point she had barely spoken a word in three years—asked the other patients to defend the woman's dignity by refusing the worker re-entry. People stood up, joined hands, and blocked the door. They let anyone out, but no one in. Two days later, in the midst of a media circus, Vera allegedly broke the human blockade to shake the mayor's hand after he personally apologized for the city worker's insult. Inspired, Vera became a peer leader. She started a patient advocacy organization and eventually joined Horizons' homeless engagement team.

PEP members would find their own recoveries by advocating for each other, as well, she hoped. In a 2006 interview, Vera shared her views on "empowerment" for PEP members:

> Empowering yourself to take back your life means exercising your freedom of choice—a fundamental right you have as an independent individual person. Empowerment has everything to do with saying "NO, that's not what I need. Don't force me or push me into something I don't want or like. Do not see me and treat me as if I were disabled. That isn't what I need from you. Let ME tell you what I need. And, for God's sake, please see me as your neighbor, family, and friend, not as a diagnosis!"

Vera hoped PEP members would gain control over their own money, "meaning they are their own payee and have their own mind and make their own decisions." She also wanted PEP members to realize, "you don't need to have anyone telling you what to do! Just do what you need to do."

"Eating anywhere"

For Vera, empowerment was contagious. She wanted to find a cause everyone could get behind that created visible change. She decided that "eating anywhere" was one such cause. Before Vera came to the center and started PEP, Riverside Club's members dined in two designated second floor areas—a small, windowless dining room, and a dining room where the air sparkled with dust illuminated by enormous latticed windows. In the larger dining area, a "recovery quilt" made of construction paper hung on one wall. Riverside members decorated each paper patch of the "quilt" to show what recovery meant to them, such as: "recovery is a rainbow" or "recovery is having food and shelter."

Members and staff volunteered to prepare, serve, and clean up a hot lunch every day. We ate at long, folding tables in red, plastic chairs. Some days we munched on tasty nacho chips with spiced ground meat, lettuce, tomato, and a few shreds of cheddar. Other days, we choked down a slab of "mystery meat" I eventually identified as Spam while volunteering in the kitchen. The milk and coffee flowed. Everyone appreciated a free, warm meal.

The clatter of forks, dishes, and trays filled the silence.

Then one day, Vera entered the larger dining hall during lunch with an entourage of PEP staff and members. She stood up on a chair.

"This is like our house!" she shouted. "We are all adults, and eating in a designated space is an institutional practice! It puts us down, right? It takes away the family feeling of taking meals together in whatever place we think is right. In your house, no one tells you to sit down and shut up and eat in the dining room, right?"

Now the members looked interested, although I thought of how many times my mother told me to eat at the kitchen table growing up.

"If the people working in this building really respect users and user choice, then they will respect us enough to let us eat wherever we want. In the business center. At the pool table. In front of the TV. Wherever! Because when we are shown the respect that we can make our own choice about where we eat, we will show it back by cleaning things up and keeping our home nice no matter where we eat. Right, guys?"

Slowly, a few members stood up, followed by more, and we streamed out of the cafeteria savoring the thrill of solidarity. We left our lame lunch trays at the table, and carried our plates casually in one hand and our milk in the other with our silverware tucked in a pocket. Riverside staff frowned, but complied on the days PEP and Riverside operated simultaneously. When PEP was not open (Monday through Wednesday), Riverside members had to eat in the designated dining areas.

Lunchtime, I noted, gained vitality. We ate while listening to the business center radio. We ate in front of the TV. We ate while we played pool. We chatted, clustered, and laughed—while eating. Some members wandered into the same chairs with the same trays to slowly eat their lunch with an even greater solitude than before.

These members may have even liked the added layer of calm in the dusty dining room.

For Vera, the important part was that everyone made a choice about where they wanted to eat. The members had been given the opportunity to act as moral agents—to make a choice that resonated with what seemed to be the common good, and so they gained confidence in their capacity to make good choices that made possible connections with others. But while they were developing their ability to act on their own for the common good, it proved to be a learning process.

No one cleaned beyond the dining area. The members had been taught to expect a janitor to clean the other spaces. And so, the inevitable happened quickly. People eating burgers next to the pool table dribbled ketchup and mustard on the floor. French fries and peas accumulated in the crevices of couches.

Vera proposed a solution. If a member saw another person leaving a mess, she could say something. "Hold each other accountable!" she encouraged. "Show some responsibility! Advocate for your rights! Defend them!"

Despite her message, people had very little experience in telling each other what to do. Smears of icing and pizza sauce appeared on armrests and keyboard keys, and trails of crumbs looped and veered across the carpet. Who was going to tell Abe to eat with his mouth closed, or ask Tessa to use a napkin instead of the arm rests?

"We have a right to be treated as adults. Demand it! Live up to it! We don't have to comply with their rules, you guys! But you need to keep it clean!" Vera insisted, but few listened.

The Business Center

Around this time, a story circulated among the members that the business center used to be the "President's Office," a former site of "member oppression." Behind the locked doors of the "President's Office," the story went, Riverside once conducted weekly staff meetings to which members were never invited, even though the activities and rules for members were debated and decided there.

The fact that members had "stormed the gates" and taken over the "office"—indeed, played games at the very table where these disempowering decisions were made—and that they had turned it into a business center to work toward independence only proved how things were changing. This was sacred—and hard earned—ground. Giving it up would reverse this victory.

Making use of this story, Vera insisted the business center door remain open at all times to empower members. The Riverside business center "volunteers" (who were also members) led by Grace (a peer and former member who had joined Riverside's staff), however, requested the door be closed for one hour each Friday. The volunteers ran the business center during the week. For some time, the volunteers had closed the door for one hour every Friday afternoon to share pizza (their own "eating anywhere" rebellion, perhaps) and assemble Riverside welcome packets. They closed the door to keep other members from coming in and messing up the packets or taking the pizza.

Vera kept opening the door, and Grace kept asking non-volunteers to leave and closing it. Vera was furious. When Grace took the next stop and *locked* the door one Friday, Vera used her staff key to burst in with a rowdy group of PEP members shouting, "Recovery! Get it, get over it, or get out!"

Tensions mounted. Grace conducted an anonymous survey of member opinions to prove everyone supported the closing of the business center for one hour on Fridays to let the volunteers assemble member packets. Vera challenged the results, which favored Grace's claim, claiming the survey did not adequately represent PEP members. The door stayed open.

Grace stopped ordering pizza so that PEP members could not take it. The volunteers dwindled, and Grace's pioneering efforts to have the members run their own business center and create welcome packets failed. On the other hand, Grace could have used a different room—there were many upstairs. Or she could have held the meeting on a day PEP was not open, which included Monday, Tuesday, and Wednesday.

The very senior administrator assigned to referee the conflict held a meeting in the business center, which Melanie also attended.

I was there as they publicly told PEP staff to stop complaining about Riverside's rules and start empowering members to advocate for the changes members actually desired. Members needed to form a consensus and initiate change, they said, rather than being told what to do by PEP staff.

In front of everyone, I piped up to put in my two cents about the member's perspective. I explained the troubled history of the room—the way it used to be the president's office and was a symbol of member exclusion. The administrator looked perplexed, but listened. As an observer privy to all of these positions, trying desperately to be neutral but finding it to be difficult, I then suggested we establish a PEP Members' Council so that members could raise and address community concerns. Riverside had a Members' Council representative that went to the AAMC meetings, so why would PEP not want representation?

The administrator listened to me, and then later that day, she and Jacob pulled me into his office. They told me it was not true—the story was a myth. The business center had never been an office; it was a library before. They said it was not a symbol of member oppression. I have no idea who was right, but felt demoralized and annoyed—did the members make that up? Did Vera? But—they added—they also agreed PEP should have representation on the members' council, and they thanked me for my time.

PEP Members' Council?

When I met with her later, Vera shrugged off the part about the business center myth, but she loved the idea of having a PEP members' council. Vocal members, she assured me, would support her changes and Riverside's clinical staff would have to respect them or risk being anti-empowerment. In her dream for PEP, everyone would be welcome to eat anywhere, the radio in the business center could play as loud as the members wanted, the executive table in the business center could be used for members to play games and socialize, and no one would pay for their afternoon snack. "Just like their own home," she said passionately (which most did not have).

Vera asked me to initiate PEP's member council so that no one could accuse her of creating a squad of toadies. She then tried to micromanage my list, but I resisted. I chose ten active and admired PEP members to create buzz and gave them a written invitation to start organizing the council on specific weekends so that Riverside would not be there (to avoid space conflicts such as those faced by Grace and her volunteers). Vera felt confident that the PEP Member's Council would make important decisions that aligned with her beliefs because she felt she knew members' hearts and minds best.

Eight out of the ten people I invited participated; the other two promised to come to the next meeting. At the first meeting, we discussed logistics. The members took a very professional approach. They would post minutes, plan agendas, and conduct elections for president, vice president, secretary, and treasurer.

But when we held an open council meeting the next week, Vera also came. It was clear that she wanted to quickly ratify her edicts. She was sure the members would support her. Instead, members giddily advocated against her.

"Empowering people is a really nice idea," Sheila began hesitantly, "but I think letting people eat anywhere is really disgusting."

"I second that," boomed Rufus. "It's just not right—all of the little crumbs everywhere and the gunk on the keyboard and phones—yuck! And I think that some of the people in here stink! Staff need to make them take a shower or tell them to leave! Isn't that what the showers are for?"

Vera piped up: "But those people don't want to take a shower, and it should be their choice not to. How are we going to show them we respect their choices if we force them to do something against their will? You, as members, need to not complain to staff. You need to talk to that member, as a member, about the value of self-care."

"I don't know 'bout you," said Dan—a lover of themed outfits like "leather" or "red, white, and blue"—"but no one wants to talk to someone who smells so bad it's nasty. How is that going to help a person be better to let them walk around in our community all nasty? No one's gonna let them be nasty out there!" He pointed out the window. "Are we not as good as them that we don't deserve to ask to be treated like normal people?"

"Yeah," boomed Rufus again, "we have to teach each other to be appropriate and part of that is hygiene. Until people can be appropriate, is it right to let them do whatever they want? They can't do that in the real world, after all."

That day, PEP's Members' Council generated ten "House Rules." Vera stomped around trying to change their minds, but this caused the members to campaign more. I quietly knitted, feeling very nervous.

Vera could have seen this as a sign that members were really learning to self-advocate, that they actually felt some moral agency in her presence and did not think self-advocating would hurt their relationship with her. Instead, she was angry that they were making rules that looked a lot like the Riverside rules she had been trying to protest. Members would eat only in the designated dining areas. The business center would be a quiet space for serious tasks. Listening to the radio would be reserved for the foyer, pool area, or art room. As for games, the dining room tables provided ample space, and the business center was not a place for play.

When it came time to enforce the rules, though, Vera forbade her PEP staff from assisting. Vera told them the new rules disempowered members. Without Vera's support, members had no moral agency to define the common good, and no power. She told them to enforce the rules themselves if they liked them so much.

"Isn't that the job of staff?" Dan demanded. "Do they not want a job?" None of the members wanted to enforce the rules, especially without any ability to reward or punish, although the idea that one of them might walk around with a walkie-talkie "just like the staff" gave some a thrill.

Without the backing of staff, PEP's Member Council became important only to the few members who earned $25 and a free sandwich as representatives of PEP to the Horizons Members' Council. This only reinforced the notion that this was all members wanted. And so, the self-fulfilling prophecy that members were not capable of recovery was reinforced.

They were right, though, members were not capable of recovery under these conditions and with these roles, rules, and relationships. A very real lack of power to enforce change at PEP—the place they thought of as their own—discouraged the members. They seemed to lose self-confidence. They also lost the ability to summon favors from peer staff. They lost the very little moral agency they had gained as new members of PEP.

This had an impact on their everyday lives. Later, when opportunities arose—say, for an apartment or a part-time job—it seemed to me that peer staff overlooked naysayers. Much like Riverside staff, PEP staff who had power, no matter how limited, continued to constrain choices for members. I could not help but think how Ella would have been disappointed if she knew how things worked behind the curtain at PEP.

Vera continued to offer snacks, sodas, and large sheet cakes on the business center's executive table most afternoons. She asked that members clean up after themselves, and they did—a little. Sometimes a PEP staff member vacuumed, but not on a schedule and not every time we ate. Riverside staff simmered.

"We can't control what they do here on the weekends," a Riverside staff member announced in a closed-door weekly staff meeting. "However, we can all avoid the upholstered chairs and couches because it's just a matter of time before we have bugs." I suddenly realized I was the only person seated on an upholstered couch with a fading, red, monkey motif. The rest of the staff sat on hard, uncomfortable, and hygienic plastic chairs they carried in from the dining area. As some glanced in my direction, my face flushed—was I embarrassed or empowered? Unsure, I remained in my seat.

The food particles eventually attracted a mouse population large enough to infest the center with mice mites. The center closed for two days of fumigation. Members had nowhere to go; unsalaried peer staff lost precious hours. My dog, who visited the center with me on the weekends, itched so furiously he needed an antibiotic. Afterward, Vera continued to serve snacks in the business center in the afternoon, but she made sure peer staff or a specific volunteer tidied up.

The great experiment in eating anywhere seemed to be a failure; however, Vera continued to claim that choosing to eat in the dining room gave members ownership, and a sense of home. Making their own rules—even if they were the same as the institutional rules that had been imposed on them before, she said—made rules feel more like choices. Oddly, the very person who encouraged the members to make their own rules ignored the rules they tried to make. PEP seemed to be making the same mistakes as Horizons.

The Greater Good

PEP's members seemed resilient, though, and continued to express their opinions to each other. Henrietta reflected: "giving people hope by giving them choices is important, but no one is going to recover if they aren't willing to make the effort. Why should people be allowed to eat anywhere if they aren't willing to clean up after themselves? That's hurting everyone else's recovery."

During an interview, Grace, the sole "out" peer provider on Riverside's staff, squinted thoughtfully up at her office ceiling. "The way I see it, there is a sense of empowerment people have gotten, and that's good and healthy," she said slowly. "But you can't have empowerment without responsibility, and what's happened here is more that of, like—I do these things. I have a right to do these things. And people do, but so does everybody else. Everyone has a right to be in a positive community setting."

She looked directly at me, as though she now felt comfortable with the sound of her own voice. "People must obey the rules of a community, not just the rules of their self. We need to respect everyone in their own recovery. Part of this is knowing that not everyone is at the point in their recovery where they should be allowed to make their own decisions, like maybe if you can't handle being a clean eater then you shouldn't be eating wherever."

Grace's comments reminded me of an Alternatives 2006 presentation during which Amy Jones, a peer provider, explained, "It's important to give members choice but it's also important that staff concerns are acknowledged. It doesn't help people if you pretend it's all about them. Living in a community—anyone's community—means it's about more than them."

Grace and Amy, in retrospect, were really talking about moral agency.

Becoming moral agents was more complicated than just taking action; it meant understanding the needs of the community and what it meant to become a community member in good standing. This required hard practice with guidance and accountability, which members rarely received. Unfortunately, seasoned, well-trained peer providers like Amy Jones (quoted earlier in the chapter) were not there to guide peer staff. Horizons also offered PEP staff little guidance.

Riverside staff continued to voice their concern. During an interview in her office, a senior staff member told me: "There's something about recovery that's scary. It's not cookie cutter and needs to be in flow. But in terms of the group, there have to be stop signs and rules to regulate traffic. You can't all be first in line. You can't all listen to the radio station you want. Where does recovery and maintaining order meet?"

Members shared these questions, but they seemed to have no voice. Even when they tried to self-advocate, members had few opportunities to make legitimate and lasting changes in the center, or at Horizons, or in society at large (Lord and Dufort 1996; Nelson, Lord, and Ochocka 2001). They had no power of their own with which to be empowered, and no capacity to obtain it without intimate relationships, good faith efforts, and a little bit of moral agency.

5

STEP THREE:
WORK FOR INTIMACY

If they're here, they are probably not in the
right mindset to have a real relationship.

—*Gus, 2006, Horizons professional staff*

R egardless of the season, Moe wore a large winter coat, a dress
shirt, and a tie. His eyes were often vacant, but when he felt in-
clined to socialize he was engaging. Moe often brought me pieces of
paper—newspaper articles about Bhutan's gross national happiness
or a clipping that described an international economic essay prize
that he hoped to win. One rainy afternoon, he presented me with
his résumé—a fragmented genealogy. It read:

- Captain, "It's Academic," American High School TV Contest
- President, High School Kiwanis, September 1962 to June 1963
- Executive Committee, [Town] Teenage Republicans
- President, [University] Young Democrats, November 1964–
  May 1965
- 104 semester hours Political Science
- Freelance Writer—June 1966 to August 1974, [Major City], US
  Publications: The Activist, American Scholar, Boston Globe,
  Commonweal, Dissent
- Independent Bookseller—September 1975 to November 1977
  Operate book search service, sell to public and dealers, and
  relate to partners and staff

- Piece work: putting sales labels on hardware (plumbing fixtures)—August 1997–May 1998
- Recycle Center—December 2001 to present, Bookkeeping, $6.50 per hour part time

What happened, I wondered, between 1977 and 1997? "Tell me about this résumé," I suggested.

"My fiancée was murdered."

Moe had been a writer, he told me, all of his life. In the late 1960s, like many young people of his time, he and his girlfriend left their home state to "tune in and drop out" in a large and fabulous city. Moe earned money writing political pieces. Sadie waitressed. They saved until they had enough money to open a small, independent bookstore. Moe knew the time was right, and he asked Sadie to marry him.

But one night in 1977, Sadie did not come home. Moe found her in a puddle of blood near the entrance of the bookstore. She had been locking up for the night, he said, when an armed thief took her life. Moe said he had a complete mental breakdown—his first ever. Losing Sadie, he claimed, triggered the psychosis that has plagued him ever since.

He had tried taking medications, but they did not work for him. He still took them and suffered immense side effects—weight gain, neurological tics that caused him to smack his lips like a fish gulping for air—but he still experienced symptoms. Moe was disabled by his voices, and now could only work part-time doing bookkeeping in the smoky back room of a small local business.

When the center was closing for the day, I offered Moe a ride. Rain fell in torrents. Moe accepted. "I am attending a community philosophy meeting," he announced, grinning widely. He clutched a dilapidated, well-tabbed copy of Heidegger's *Being and Time*.

"Oh, that's exciting," I said. "Is this a member group?" Moe had run a happiness group for members at Horizons that I had attended, which is where we met.

"Oh, no," Moe beamed. "These are real, normal people! People from the community. About ten."

"Really?"

"Mostly young people. We meet once a week so I can teach them. This week I will teach them about Heidegger."

"How did you meet them?"

"I put a free ad in the paper asking if anyone wanted to start a philosophy group—and they all came!"

"Cool. How long have you been going?"

"A couple of times."

As I watched him disappear behind the fogged glass door of the coffee shop, I smiled. How nice, I thought, he was finally connecting with people who appreciated him.

A few weeks later, Moe and I were sharing coffee again, and I asked how his meeting went. He fumbled with his foam cup.

"Well, you know where you dropped me off?" he asked.

"I do."

"They weren't there," he croaked.

"Oh."

Moe peered up at me over his crooked, wire glasses, "I put another advertisement in the paper asking where people went, but . . ."

As far as Moe and I know, no one came again.

Earlier in the year, Moe had led a Happiness Group with a clinic staff member at a smoky local diner, which I also attended. Many of the attendees, fellow users of the mental health clinic, seemed to enjoy the group. But when he tried to translate that success into the community by starting a community philosophy group—a group with people he thought of as "normal"—they came a few times, and then stopped coming.

It is impossible to say why the entire group decided to stop coming, but this kind of scenario is not isolated to Moe's life. It's a storyline that I have seen play out again and again as I have tried to investigate ethnographically the lives of people diagnosed with serious mental illnesses in the United States. In his effort to recover, Moe tried to publicly craft himself as a quirky philosopher on a quest for happiness, but other people did not recognize him as such. Maybe it had nothing to do with him, but he took it personally. He felt demoralized and lonely.

He could secure intimate connections with people inside the center, but would he ever find them "out there?" Finding one's niche in the community, as Davidson (2009:44) and colleagues advised people in recovery to do, proved difficult. Out there, if you were unemployed, poor, and strange, people were not just going to offer you the benefit of the doubt that you were a moral person worthy of an intimate relationship. As Horizons' recovery philosophy seemed to plainly state, you had to earn it. You had to become a hard-working, taxpaying citizen. Without this springboard to moral belonging, it was hard to act in a way that resonated with others. Most of the members who were serious about recovery and had not resigned themselves to being "regulars" at Horizons thus spent most of their time trying to position themselves to find meaningful work—and keep it.

Recovery as Gainful Employment

The whole enterprise of recovery at Horizons aimed to put people back to work. The absence of moral regard from people "out there" had much to do with members' unemployment status—and all that preceded this inability upstream, and all that flowed from it. In US culture, what is most important (i.e., moral) is to participate in the social contract by working hard to secure a better future for all (Nussbaum 2006). Never mind Marxist readings of "work" as the product of a subjugated person who is alienated from their labor. Most members and recovery advocates, fully immersed in American neoliberal ideals, never mentioned anything along those lines. They all wanted the members to be gainfully employed. As recovery leader Joseph Rogers (schizophrenia.com 2005) noted, "although people need help with their emotional problems, if they don't have some way to make a living they will never truly be able to enter, or re-enter the mainstream." Assisting people with finding work "might be the most useful role [mental health clinicians] could play in the lives of people who want a piece of the American dream."

Similarly, Jacobson and Greenley (2001:483) wrote that finding connection in recovery came through finding roles one could play in the world, preferably roles that would benefit others as well as oneself. This could all be thought of as the "work of recovery," a process through which people learned to "take back control" of their own lives, privately and publicly (Davidson et al. 2009:61).

Employment was understood to be a main facilitator of recovery, and many people in recovery expressed a desire to work (Davidson et al. 2009:45). Gainful employment assuaged symptoms, aided in the building of interpersonal relationships, and increased user perceptions that one lived a "good" life (Baron 1995; Bell and Lysaker 1997; O'Day and Killeen 2002; Rutman 1994). Without a job, however, Horizons members like Moe had difficulty participating in the moral order "out there." Without work, how could they recover?

Recognizing the need for more competitive employment opportunities for service users, recovery advocates often suggest users find meaningful work *within* the mental health care system (Dixon, Krauss, and Lehman 1994; Medscape 2005; Van Tosh 1993). Being a peer provider helped him, Joseph Rogers explained, because he realized "I could not only receive help but could give it" (schizophrenia.com 2005). Vera said something similar about her own work. Recovery proponents claimed that "anyone could work," and that everyone had a right to a meaningful job (paid or not) regardless of their level of disability (DHHS 2003b).

Members I knew often desired paid employment. Some volunteered, hoping to improve and establish their utility. Some volunteered in the kitchen, or supervised and cleaned the private bathroom, clothing closet (of donated clothes), and laundry room used by homeless members, or offered technical assistance with computers in the business center. Vera invited PEP members to start their own "recovery classes." Vlad once ran a chess and checkers group, for example, and Sheila ran the highly successful relationships group for eight months until Vera made her a staff member.

A lucky few at the center, like Sheila, did "move up" to receive stable, part-time, minimum-wage positions (with no benefits) as a peer specialist. Members who became employees typically desired to work part-time to avoid reductions in their disability-related government benefits, including their monthly stipends and medical insurance. Maintaining one's benefits provided a safety net. I saw only one recovery worker at the center, Luke, let go of his benefits and shift into a competitive, full-time position.

Opportunities outside the center were much more rare. I knew one long-standing Riverside member who volunteered at a zoo. A few people I knew also found volunteer jobs (or minimum-wage, part-time jobs) as recovery facilitators at local hospital inpatient programs. All were efforts to establish members' capacities to become wage-earning, moral agents in a society where moral worth was often based on one's ability to contribute to the economic future of all. In order to be a welcome member of the broader community, a person had to work. But in order to work, a person had to know how to be a good worker. In order to know how to be a good worker, a person needed to be accountable, and they needed meaningful relationships—caring, intimate relationships—to learn how to do this.

Earning recognition and moral regard "in here" at Horizons, in contrast, created something of a paradox. In general, as service users increasingly participated in mental health programs and moved away from working, they reported fewer social ties with less diversity and reciprocity in their relationships and felt less satisfied and more lonely than their peers (Angell 2003). The moral regard members cultivated at Horizons, I found, aside from not gaining them much traction within Horizons, also did not seem to translate into moral agency in the outside community, and they lacked the intimate relationships with coworkers, family, lovers, and so forth, that they needed to replenish their moral agency in the first place.

Recovery Workers

Even so, many PEP members admired Horizons employees and aspired to become one. They seemed to be exemplars of everything that was "good" at Horizons. Members imagined that being a Horizons staff member also translated into moral recognition outside the center.

"Horizons is the best," one member told me, "and they have helped me to do my best, so why wouldn't I want to work for the best?" Being one of the best, the members thought, surely earned one respect in the community-at-large.

Recovery advocates heavily promoted the idea that "recovered" users deserved gainful employment in the mental health system due to their acquired expertise successfully navigating the system and managing their symptoms (Boykin 1997; DHHS 2003a; Dixon, Kraus, and Lehman 1994; Mowbray et al. 1996; Solomon and Draine 2001). Six out of eleven of Vera's peer providers were members-turned-recovery workers. Some were early members of PEP who did so well that Vera made them staff. According to the research, the peer staff's acquired expertise as former members made them effective role models and advisers (Boykin 1997; Dixon, Kraus, and Lehman 1994; Solomon and Draine 1996).

One of the members, Damien, explained the effect of having positive role models:

> When you live at the nursing home, you see the other nursing home people, and you see them come in, and they're struggling to just walk down the hallway, and you know they can't work, and you're there, too, so you can't work. Me, deep inside, I never thought I could work again. But then you come in here, and you think—wow, maybe in a while longer I could do this, too. So how do I go about trying to do this?

Peer provider Thelma had a similar sentiment:

> I think they come in and they see us, and they say—wow, you have a job. I think everybody, and I don't care how lazy they are, they think, "Oh I never want to work again." But then they realize they want to do something. Everybody likes to do something. And they look at us and think, "They're doing something and they're good at it and they're making money. And it's good because it will help others."

At the center, at least one PEP staff member could probably serve as an effective role model for almost anyone who walked through the door. PEP staff consistently disclosed their struggles to members. Every peer staff member had experience with homelessness, mental health treatment, and hospitalization. They accentuated commonalities between themselves and members in hopes of forming a trusting and inspirational relationship.

"Recovered" psychiatrist Dan Fisher explained the value of this practice in a 2004 lecture at a National Association for Rights and Protection Advocacy conference: "A misapprehension of a newly-diagnosed person might initially be: 'I have a permanent condition, and I'll never recover from it.' Having another person around you who can help you understand through their life that other people have been through it and you're not alone plays a huge role in shifting that misperception to a new understanding."

During enrollment interviews with PEP, I watched many frightened initiates relax as they mutually shared struggles with trauma, substance use, sexual abuse, suicide, prison time, poverty, homelessness, and symptom or medication experiences with the PEP staff. Storytelling, research suggested, helped peer providers serve their clients well (Boykin 1997). This element of peer-based care has been referred to as "shared humanness" (Ware, Tugenberg, and Dickey 2004).

Even though PEP valued a community of shared narrative between members, this level of transparency was not for everyone. Twenty-something Jaime, for example, stopped attending PEP after a stable, six-month membership. The members told me that a member of the peer staff had spoken openly to another member about Jaime's history of "sucking dick for heroin." When asked, the accused peer provider told me that she selectively told a newcomer with a similar history Jaime's story in hopes that Jaime's recent successes—sobriety and renouncing prostitution—would inspire the new member to do the same. Jaime was furious.

When I asked the peer provider why she thought it was okay to disclose Jaime's confidential story, she said: "Peers talk to each other different. It's important that Jaime not be ashamed. It's between peers. We're peers, so we don't keep secrets from each other." Jaime, who only returned once over the next year to collect a disability stipend—belligerent and high—probably would not agree.

Professional Boundaries

Even so, the ways PEP staff shared stories contrasted with the approach of Riverside. As with many traditional psychosocial rehabilitation programs, personal information did not flow between Riverside staff and their clients (Bellah et al. 1996; Ware, Tugenberg, and Dickey 2004). Clinical staff's withholding of their own histories led some users to feel stigmatized or rejected.

"I know she has a drinking problem," one Riverside member said of his case manager after she kept calling in sick to work. "So why won't she tell me? I may be nuts, but I've been a recovered alcoholic for ten years! I could help her, but I am not good enough to help her, I guess. She is only good enough to help me."

Weekly Riverside staff meetings increased the narrative inequality between staff and clients. At these meetings, Riverside staff openly discussed members' lives in detail (behind closed doors), including histories of imprisonment, homelessness, drug abuse, sexual abuse, and their diagnoses. Riverside shared details of each member's story. Sometimes, they joked about these stories as in this moment:

> FEMALE STAFF: So Dara Banks is twenty-six, female, unmarried, diagnosis of bipolar disorder, said she drinks a lot and may have a drinking problem, no friends or family in the area.
> MALE STAFF: Oh no? Does she have a bartender? [General laughter]

Such behavior signals a disrespect that may not be heard by members so much as it is felt. It also widens the gulf between two people and prevents them from developing a position of solidarity between them. Staff and client may become estranged, even in the midst of great one-way intimacy.

One morning, for example, Horace gave Elizabeth, his Riverside case manager, an office plant for her birthday. "Elizabeth has been my case manager for ten years," he told me at lunch, looking very pleased. "So I saved up spare change to buy her an office plant. She's really been there for me."

This meant a lot to Horace. As we know, he never felt supported by his family.

"Did she like it?" I asked.

"I think she liked it," he said, "but she never shows her feelings very well." As we ate, Horace looked increasingly worried.

"Maybe she didn't like it," he fretted. "Or maybe she didn't want people to know it was her birthday."

"I am sure it's fine," I told him.

Later that afternoon, I ducked into Elizabeth's office to wish her a happy birthday. A lovely, white Easter Lilly stood on the windowsill. Elizabeth waved me in, shut the door, and began to whisper:

Look at this plant! Horace knows he's not supposed to do that! It's not allowed. Now what am I supposed to do? I don't want the stupid plant but if it's not in my office he's going to be offended, and spend the whole time whining about it. And if I accept it, then our relationship changes. I break the rule, and he thinks I am breaking it because he's special. And then who knows where he'll go with that one?

Elizabeth wanted her relationship with Horace to remain clinical. Powerful institutional rules—known as "clinical boundaries"—shaped traditional relationships between staff and clients. Clinical boundaries asked case managers to meet their clients at specific places and times, not to share their own life stories with users, and to refrain from exchanging gifts. But Elizabeth meant more to Horace. They had known each other for ten years. She knew everything about him. He viewed her as one of his few "normal" friends. In traditional mental health settings, the stable relationships readily available to service users like Horace were often isolated to paid, clinical staff like Elizabeth.

Over time, institutional rules had made these relationships more and more bounded—and less and less intimate. As Jacob, Riverside's program director, explained:

JACOB: Early on, the boundaries were more blurry. Staff actually hung out with members.

ME: Outside?

JACOB: Yeah, like you'd go to a game and bring members along.

ME: Okay! That does sound different.

JACOB: There wasn't that much—it was kind of like post sixties, seventies—so it hadn't got into what was clinical. Back then, you couldn't get fired as long as you didn't have sex with a member, but anything short of that there wasn't a lot of discussion. So it was comfortable, very relaxed. But somewhere between the mid-eighties, early nineties, it began to change. . . . The X generation came out, and I saw more people coming to interview for jobs that were like, "Okay, what's in it for me?" They were less humanitarian, and more of a job. Pay at a certain rate. And so, the clinical edge was very "What's in it for me? We aren't friends. I am just getting paid to be your friend. Oh, and how much will I be paid?"

In a separate conversation, a thirty-something Riverside staff member, Chris, discussed his perspective on clinical boundaries. Chris thought boundaries were crucial to his successes:

Not to be mean, but I don't want to share my life with them. I am not inviting them to my house. I want them to stay here when I leave. They are work. As long as they depend on us for companionship, they are never going to be completely independent of us and that's not healthy. Part of recovery is having friends who aren't paid friends.

"When Chris is out of town or absent," one of his bosses told me later, "it's like the phone line's been cut for these members. They don't even talk to us." The mental image of a ruptured phone line, or a busy signal, reinforced my sense of how tenuous clinical relationships were for members, how much they depended on staff for connectedness, and how easy—and desirable—it was for staff to ignore that connection.

Limitations to intimacy are found everywhere—from the workplace (no intimacy between coworkers or bosses and their underlings) to educational settings (no relationships between teachers or professors and their students). Boundaries seemingly protect the less powerful party in the relationship (the student, the mental health client, the worker hoping for a promotion) from exploitation. Clinicians like Chris and Elizabeth erected clinical boundaries to help clients be "more healthy in their relationships" and "independent." Case workers also desired to maintain separate lives outside of "work."

According to these rules, they could ignore a patient if they bumped into each other at the pharmacy. They could "cut the phone line" and take a vacation if needed. But these boundaries put members in a challenging position. Can one build one's capacities to engage in intimate relationships without being able to summon the relationships one needs to learn how to be in relationships?

Intimate Workers

Peer services intended to help users develop social networks that would enable them to practice being good friends and workers (Solomon and Draine 2001). Advocates claimed that nurturing peer environments would emphasize "strengths over weaknesses, people over labels, lives over cases—and the idea and the belief that lives can be transformed for the better, not as a matter of charity and pity, but as a matter of principle, love, respect, and reason" (Pierce 2004:404). These founding principles, supporters of peer services believed, could best be upheld by peer providers because peers worked *with* users, rather than *for* users (Mead and Copeland 2000:6). As Fisher and Chamberlin (2004:5) explained, "we have taken people out of the institutions, but we haven't taken the institutional thinking out of people." Peer services aimed to correct institutional thinking, which limited intimacy between users and the providers because peers were often one of the few resources members had for learning how to act locally as a moral agent.

In one key move to cast off institutional thinking, PEP expected peer providers to reject clinical boundaries. As we have seen, Riverside staff (as with most traditional case managers) met users at a specific time and place, kept personal information shared with users to a minimum, avoided interacting with users outside of treatment, and refused to accept gifts (Ware, Tugenberg, and Dickey 2004). Members like Horace, Davidson and colleagues (2009:163) wrote, eventually became "accustomed to having their offers of reciprocity rejected because traditional client-clinician therapeutic boundaries and roles forbid such a two-way street." But members needed to develop their capabilities to cultivate outside friendships and find good jobs. Horace needed Elizabeth to accept his gift AND insist on a mutually comfortable relationship so that Horace could practice what that meant.

At PEP, Vera and her staff tinkered with clinical boundaries to create an allegedly egalitarian environment. An egalitarian environment, advocates thought, would provide empowerment, autonomy, and hope for individuals rather than paternalistic, degrading directives for care (Buchannan 2008; Jacobson 2004; SAMHSA 2006). Aligning with these principles, the PEP Vision Statement claimed, "there is genuine equality and all are equal to revise anything about [PEP] or what it offers." Vera presented PEP as a place where people "who have no other support can go for socializing and kindness offered by each other and by people with similar experiences of the pain, suffering, embarrassment, and rejection that comes from having mental illness, substance abuse and homelessness."

To reduce clinical boundaries, for example, PEP had a "no-appointment policy." Anyone should be able to talk to any staff member at any time, Vera insisted. Appointments reinforced hierarchies. In theory, members could access peer staff any time the center was open. But members often waited an hour or more to catch PEP staff between activities. With four regular peer staff serving ten to sixty people each day, obtaining assistance could be confusing. When peer staff took a sick day, the situation became chaotic. The policy also made it difficult for PEP staff to schedule personal needs, such as lunch, or a bathroom or smoke break, into an unstructured day.

When PEP staff met with members in community settings, they made appointments, but staff did not always keep them. Irate members met with landlords and navigated the social security office alone. Members perceived these practices as disrespectful.

"It's like my time doesn't matter to them," Harlem said. "That's some serious disrespect."

"Along with the lack of appointments," Marigold fumed, "comes a lack of commitment!"

Harlem and many others discontinued their enrollment in PEP in favor of Riverside or other services in the city, they claimed, for this specific reason.

Peer staff also managed the "gifts boundary" differently than Riverside staff like Elizabeth. Vera accepted "paper gifts" like cards or drawings and indirectly gave members gifts at group events.

"What's a birthday without a cake and some gifts?" Vera asked me.

At these parties, we all signed a card with a ten dollar bill slipped into it from "all of us." On holidays, Vera had "special" rounds of Bingo with donated wrapped presents. Vera also handed out coupons she found for free drinks or fries. These practices loosened—but did not eliminate—boundaries despite Vera's egalitarian claims.

On several occasions the members offered me presents, which I hesitantly accepted. Members gave me drawings, cards, artwork, and poems. Henrietta brought me used makeup because she was concerned about my drab appearance. Another woman gave me homemade jewelry. Despite my protests, if we went out of the center for a cup of coffee, the member often insisted on paying. When the members threw me a baby shower, about twenty people gave me presents ranging from gift cards to diapers and bundles of baby clothes. It strengthened our sense of togetherness. This was a very moving experience, but accepting one gift meant accepting them all. Members competed over the gifts they gave me. "I bought her coffee" would be followed by "Well, I gave her a necklace which she will keep forever."

I did not give anyone tangible gifts as the need was so great, but I offered them my time, attention, and energy. Since I was not a "paid friend" and did this for free, my efforts—however staff-like—did not cross professional boundaries, but offered members what some have called "social dignity," or the socially-negotiated messages conveyed by interpersonal interactions about one's worth (Jacobson, Oliver, and Koch 2009). These messages, while social, also shaped one's self-regard. Dignity violation was more likely to occur in non-egalitarian situations where one actor was vulnerable (in this case, the members) and the other subject to antipathy (e.g., staff). In contrast, I shared with members a certain solidarity, which Jacobson and colleagues (2009) found less likely to result in a dignity violation. Peer staff had potential for developing this kind of solidarity with members, but could they alter the deeply hierarchical practices of the center's institutional culture in which PEP was embedded?

Medical Necessity

As I was leaving the field, new state-imposed Fee for Service and Medicaid billing rules began to curtail even the tentative, hard-earned intimacies being developed between members and recovery-oriented case managers—peer and professional.

"Fee for service is killing recovery," one administrator wrote to me in an email in 2010.

Under the new system, at the end of each day, staff had to spend hours filling out billing paperwork to document how every fifteen minutes they spent with a member correlated with a specific service that addressed a specific "deficit." They used a software program to open a member's file, specified how much time they spent with them, selected a service from a drop-down list and a deficit from a drop-down list, and then took notes on how that service was leading to some change in the member's mental health status. In this system, there was little room to improvise, and consistent reminders to focus on the member's weaknesses.

As the administrator explained:

> The documentation requirement that you have to show medical necessity for each fifteen-minute increment changes the thinking of the staff who provide the services. It takes extraordinary sophistication for a staff person to be thinking about empowerment, dignity of risk, strengths, goals, etc., and then to shift gears and talk about the deficit that was addressed when documenting that service. . . . I feel like Horizons is really trying to change our culture and to make everything we do more recovery oriented. However, staff often report that they're getting a mixed message. Because *they are* getting a mixed message. Document the deficits, hit your billing targets. Oh, and by the way, use a recovery approach. They just don't jibe.

Service providers across the country in states who are adopting this medical billing model are also struggling with the paradigm of "medical necessity." Agencies, for example, must deny consumers services if they are doing well. As I was leaving the field, this had only begun to occur at Horizons.

"Everyone acts like it's so bad," Dolores rolled her eyes dramatically, "that I still come here. I have had my own place for twenty years. I do volunteer work on a psychiatric ward helping other people think about recovery. I am very happy! But I still come here. I just like the people here; that's all. They've been my friends for twenty years. So I come here twice a week for company. Is that so bad?"

Gary was in a similar situation. He had his own apartment, a roommate, and a part-time job washing dishes in a cafeteria with coworkers he adored. He had not been hospitalized for years. "Still, people can tell I am a bit odd," he chuckled nervously, "especially women." He continued:

> They just kind of look at me odd. So I come here. I feel connected here. The pretty lady case managers smile at me here and ask me

how I am doing. If that makes me not recovered, then fine! If recovery is my choice, then I can choose to not recover because if I leave here I would be lonely with no women's smiles, and then I wouldn't maybe be able to go to work and relapse.

Under the rules enacted after my time at Horizons, the administrator told me, Delores and Gary were no longer welcome at the center. They had value to the center if they were "billable," but if no one could bill a fee for a service rendered, then they had no right to come. In fact, if they did, they would be asked to leave. And while policy recommendations claimed we should encourage members to "graduate" with "concrete steps being taken by the treatment team and individual toward this goal" (Davidson, et al., 2009:137), it also remained unclear how Delores and Gary were going to see their friends once they were forced to leave. I could not find Maison because I was not a family member; how would they find people or keep track of each other?

It also remained unclear how they might acquire new friends "out there." When Moe tried to make this shift by creating the community philosophy group, he was soundly rejected. He came back to the center, feelings hurt, and reminded himself that even if he could not find a niche for him in the community, he had good friends who cared for him regardless. Under the new fee-for-service rules, the administrator told me, Moe also could not use the center to socialize, although he could come in to discuss medications or pick up his disability check. Horizons' recovery model held that he needed to learn to stay well on his own. Even national-level advocates insisted on some kind of "graduation" and "exit strategy" so that services and practitioners would "not remain central to a person's life over time" (Davidson et al. 2009:137). Well, what if it has been a long time, and that is all people have?

In an interview, Melanie articulated the importance of relationships for members for me: "Be present! The whole notion of being present with people and bringing yourself with you and appreciating other selves that you encounter is an important thing for members to work on." I wish I had thought to ask her—whom are members going to work on this with if their peers are not feeling well, the outside community will not welcome them, and staff maintain strong clinical boundaries and limit everyday interactions to those that are medically necessary?

The Necessity of Intimacy

In tune with this need for practicing intimacy and relationships, PEP encouraged members to mingle. Vera consistently linked newcomers to experienced members on their first visit. We had parties to celebrate members' life events—birthdays, new jobs, getting out of a nursing home, holidays. At the parties, there were special Bingo prizes, music, dancing, and sheet cakes. PEP also opened on major holidays (Thanksgiving Day, Christmas Day, Easter Sunday) when every other mental health facility remained closed. On New Year's Eve 2006, for example, Isaac kept the center open until after midnight while twelve elated members rang in the New Year together.

Vera also lifted physical restrictions on the exchange of bodily contact between staff and members. The "Golden Rule" remained in place—staff could not date members. She encouraged hugs, having arms around each other, prolonged handholding, and pats on the shoulder, however. For example, Arthur frequently almost-kissed the hands of women who had to laughingly, but firmly, extract their hand from his.

"Oh, but he's harmless," they would chuckle. As a fellow target, I admit that he seemed harmless, and never proved to be more than harmless. I accepted his gesture as a sign of affection. If a member took things "too far," of course, boundaries were set up to help them understand how to interact in a way that made everyone comfortable. One woman, for example, was told that she would be banned for sexual harassment if she continued to grope male members. She respected their request and no longer crossed this boundary.

Vera also tried to connect members for "fun and dating." PEP offered a popular relationships class once each week. Many members discussed the challenges of presenting a history of sexual trauma in a new romantic relationship, or the complications of dating another person with psychiatric disabilities, or the terror of disclosing a mental illness to a "normal" partner. This forum brought people together to flirt, laugh, and work through difficulties with intimate relationships.

After relationships group, Vera held a "mixer" in the same room. The well-attended event often felt like a junior high dance with snacks, eighties music, and people dancing in small groups. We all laughed and grooved and had a good time.

Vera often mentioned the "taboo topic" of sex for members and angrily pointed out the discomfort clinical staff experienced when members were intimate. The Riverside staff, for example, explicitly forbade member intimacy. "If they can't even take care of themselves," one case manager asked me, "how are they supposed to be in a relationship and help care for someone else?"

Discomfort with the sexuality of people with psychiatric disabilities has long existed. Its darkest hour came during a program of forced sterilization in state hospitals, eventually condemned as a Nazi doctrine (Grob 1994; Shorter 1997:141, 161). Today, most mental health programs discourage user relationships and forbid open displays of affection. This is a travesty. As Davidson and colleagues (2009:69) wrote, "it is unreasonable and unethical to insist that a person with paraplegia regain his or her mobility in order to live independently . . . [and] it is both unreasonable and unethical to insist that a person with a serious mental illness no longer experience symptoms or have functional impairments in order to have sex."

Vera, using more of the approach of Davidson and colleagues (2009), vocalized members' desperate need for touch and affection. She encouraged intimate gestures. Ralph and Rose often rebelliously kissed—a sweet peck—in front of other members. But even as Vera applauded their happiness and their respectful display of affection, the Riverside staff requested they refrain from any sign of intimacy, including holding hands. Since Rose was originally a member of Riverside, this pressure was particularly effective. The Riverside staff were like "old friends," Rose said. Even so, Rose felt she was an adult and ought to be able to make her own decisions.

When asked about Ralph's relationship with Rose, another Riverside staff member sighed heavily. "I kind of am disappointed. I mean, I just think she would be better off with someone who was not mentally ill, too. How hard is that? Having to deal with yourself being sick and then the stress of your partner being sick, too?"

Another remarked, "If they're here, they are probably not in the right mindset to have a real relationship." Riverside staff worried, some explained, that "appropriate" affection would lead to "inappropriate affection" and disrupt the order in the milieu.

In contrast, it seemed that most members feared being alone. Many had lost custody of their children at some point. Few could afford a pet. Most people were estranged from their families. And nearly everyone longed for a little affection.

PEP was one of the few places I have seen where service users could practice intimacy before they proved that they were "in recovery" (in this context, gainfully employed). Members needed this practice to make it in the world "out there," but they had very few places to practice. New mental health policies that limit service visits to those of "medical necessity" will offer them even less.

RECOVERY'S EDGE

So much competition isn't right in a
family. Can't we all just get along?

—*Trey, 2006, PEP member*

There was too much pressure on
him. Pressure at work.

—*Sheila, 2006, PEP member
turned peer service provider*

O ne evening, as I descended the massive spiral staircase into the
central foyer, I overheard a new member screaming at Isaac. I
peered over the railing.

"LIAR! You're no different! You're just like the rest of them—you
liar! Liar!" the member, Raoul, shouted.

"Raoul has anger issues," a Riverside staff member told me the
next day, "and was very sensitive. Really at the low point for himself
in terms of symptoms and well-being."

The day before, the staff member said, Riverside's goal was to
keep Raoul calm while they decided if they should enroll him as
a new member or send him elsewhere. Around lunchtime, Raoul
needed to make a phone call, but all of the Riverside phones were in
use. A Riverside case manager, Chris, unlocked Isaac's office door to
enable Raoul to use a PEP phone—a common practice. Raoul then
demanded to take a book he found while in the office, but Chris
told Raoul he needed to ask Isaac's permission.

The rest of the day, Raoul repeatedly interrupted Isaac asking if he could borrow his book. Isaac was very busy—and this wasn't even a PEP client, Isaac later pointed out—so he told him they could talk about it later. Late in the afternoon, Raoul spotted Isaac as he was leaving for the night.

Raoul asked for the book again. Isaac said they could discuss it in the morning. Some professional staff said this proved that Isaac was on a power trip. Isaac claimed he just wanted to go home.

At this particular time, Isaac was working more and more hours with less and less support. Vera took a good deal of medical leave. Melanie, who held staff supervision meetings with the PEP staff once per week, was also on medical leave and resigned a few months later. PEP hired, trained, and then quickly lost a staff member when he relapsed on crack. Next, Vera hired Sheila, the PEP member who ran the relationships group and was president of the PEP Members' Council, but Sheila also needed training. Isaac was the only staff member prepared to run PEP.

Over time, his patience flagged. On this particular evening, his patience had run out.

"I will let you see the book tomorrow," I saw him tell Raoul calmly again, "but I have an appointment and need to go home."

The intensity skyrocketed as Raoul stepped closer to Isaac and shouted: "Nigger! You're just a stupid nigger! You have no right to say no to me!"

I am not sure who lunged first. Isaac mirrored Raoul's menacing stance, and then they collided. Isaac later claimed he had noticed the pencil Raoul had in his hand, which Raoul tried to jab into his neck. To "disarm him," Isaac grabbed Raoul's arms, twisted until he dropped the pencil, and then locked his hands behind his back. The members cleared the way.

But Isaac, who was decades older, began to lose stamina. Raoul resisted, slamming Isaac backward against a wall.

The spectators froze. Joel, the only other PEP staffer on site, emerged from the back office to survey the scene.

"Help! Somebody help me! Help!" Isaac shrieked. A burly middle-aged member stepped forward, but Jacob, the Riverside Program Director, intervened.

"Don't! Don't!" Jacob shouted. Jacob later explained that there "could have been a riot" if members stepped in. Instead of physically helping Isaac, Jacob started talking.

"Man, Raoul! Are you okay? Tell me what's going on here! And Isaac," he added sharply, "you need to let him go." At this point, other Riverside staff herded the rest of us out of sight.

"Fuel on a fire"

I sat with Isaac the morning after his "incident." "They did not have my back," Isaac stated miserably, eyes watering. He meant the Riverside staff who had handled the situation, and he thought it might be because he was black or a peer or both. We had just been at the Alternatives conference—and Isaac had moved from the heights of recovery seeing Priscilla Ridgway to a devastating low in just six weeks.

Other PEP staff were not so sure.

"He could have just offered Raoul the book," Bella observed. "No need to get killed over it." Joel characteristically raised his eyebrows, shrugged, and threw his hands in the air.

The Riverside staff plainly thought Isaac's interactions with Raoul were out of line. One staff member threatened to call the state's Solicitor General and report Isaac. "As professionals, we are trained to practice nonviolent interventions," this particular Riverside staff member told me tersely in a private interview the next day.

The person continued:

Isaac threw fuel on a fire when he grabbed Raoul! Fuel on a fire! He should have seen that pencil coming, and been down on his knees in the fetal position, begging for Raoul to calm down. "I am so sorry if I offended you! What can I do to help you?" We all know that; we learned it in our training—nonviolent intervention. In that situation, you do anything you can to help a person realize that they are being violent and talk them out of it. What Isaac did was abusive. It's just another example of how peers abuse their clients. If Raoul had actually hurt Isaac with that pencil, he could go to jail the rest of his life, all because Isaac triggered him to be more aggressive instead of doing anything he could to calm him down. I feel like I need to report Isaac for abusing a member. Isaac *abused* a member, and he is allowed to be at work today!

Horizons never trained Isaac—a combat veteran—in nonviolent intervention, though.[1] If this was a basic safety standard, why was training in "Crisis Management and Response" not part of Isaac's mandatory orientation as it had been for Riverside staff? PEP's off-site supervisor told me that training would not have made a difference. Isaac did not punch Raoul, the person said, he reacted like the soldier he had been. I responded that it might have made a difference, and we cannot know for sure; now, it is too late.

Vera thought Isaac's interactional style stemmed from his previous institutional experiences. He put a member in restraints—much like an orderly in a mental hospital, she said—because the same had been done to him. Vera observed, "Some of us feel like we have to prove ourselves, and we're pissed off about the way we were treated. . . . We were pushed around and told we weren't as good as them. Anger is our energy."

Open Door?

Institutional factors also fed into Isaac's incident. In the two years prior (2004 through 2006), the demographics at Horizons' Recovery Center had changed. Riverside's "regulars" blamed PEP for the change, but around the same time PEP opened, Riverside commenced an "open door" policy. Sometimes, Riverside and PEP waited a couple of weeks to "intake" a new member and collect their personal history and insurance information. Riverside said they wanted newcomers to feel comfortable, and this practice reduced their paperwork burden when prospective members left after a week or two.

A Riverside staff member explained the policy shift:

> In the twenty-five years I have been here, it's only been in the last two years that we have had homeless people in the program. Before we really creamed the best off the top and screened people. And now that we are letting them in, I am wondering—oh, my God, where are the resources for these homeless people? Or, why are they declining places [housing] for this reason or that reason?

Between the open-door policy and the intake delay, unsavory characters sometimes roamed the center. Some Riverside staff fretted over safety concerns. "There's a volatility. Every once in a while, there is a tension in the lobby, or around the pool table, that is too intense."

Another Riverside staff member defended both the open-door policy and PEP:

> ME: What made the milieu at the center feel less safe?
> RS: Well, even before [PEP] came here we started having the homeless come in—
> ME: Why do you mention them? Was the center not unsafe before the open-door policy?
> RS: It was unsafe before. It's not true. It's not the homeless' fault. . . . You can blame it on me. It's the open door policy, and I pushed for it to happen. Word got out on the street, and people just started walking in, and that's the way it should be: an open door.
> ME: I've heard people say it used to be so peaceful, quiet . . .
> RS: They need to get over that. I am with Vera. We work for the chronic mentally ill. Vera and I actually agree on a lot of things. She just doesn't know it.

Whatever the cause, everyone agreed the center had changed. A sharp increase in theft prompted suspicions. Members reported sketchy characters following them as they left in the evening. Some were agitated by the confusion and fear in the milieu. Gary and I were eating lunch when he told me, "It's not right, the riff-raff being in here. They shouldn't be allowed. This is a place for getting better, not an indoor street corner."

Entrenched Riverside staff voiced anxieties:

> The milieu right now is out of control. I have members coming in my office telling me it's out of control, and something bad is going to happen. People are swearing, angry, about to get in fights. People telling me that everything is angry on the weekends [when PEP is the only place open]. You feel like you're being pushed, like people make snide comments at you. Are there the same people here on the weekends as during the week because it's the same names?

These allegations of weekend chaos surprised me. I spent most weekends at PEP (open between nine a.m. and four p.m. Thursday through Sunday) and found it to be more peaceful when Riverside did not operate concurrently. Dealing with thirty to forty members instead of one hundred and fifty members relaxed everyone, and the center seemed more like a house. People chatted, used the computers, lounged, read the paper, played games, and enjoyed each other's company. There were few rules, but few conflicts or incidents. To me, this seemed the opposite of chaos.

Without witnessing this personally, some Riverside staff persisted with their hunch that PEP had a negative influence on members. The members, one Riverside staffer complained, "come running to tattle to Riverside whenever PEP does something wrong, but we're powerless to do anything about it! But if PEP messes something up, well, then we're welcome to pick up the slack for them. They have no problems taking our help, but they never take our advice."

Members longed for peace.

"So much competition isn't right in a family," Trey told me, "can't we all just get along?"

Members accepted that PEP and Riverside met different needs. They tried to bridge the rift by joining the Riverside Members' Council with PEP's Members' Council, but a squabble over potential office space in the flood-prone basement derailed them. One PEP member allegedly told a Riverside member that they could not locate the planned Riverside Members' Council office in the basement because "everyone knows the basement is for PEP." While untrue, PEP was the only program making official use of the basement where they had set up the clothing closet, the laundry room, and a private bathroom.

Offended, Riverside's Member's Council ceased collaborative efforts. PEP members claimed they had merely been asking whether they could share the office when Riverside insisted it was theirs. "I wonder sometimes," one member told me quietly, "if this place has any adults in it!"

"It wore us all out."

Apparently not long after I left the field (six weeks after Isaac clashed with Raoul), Isaac had a mental health and substance abuse relapse. He went from being well on the way to recovery back to being hospitalized and unemployed. The incident with Raoul, the absence of Vera and Melanie, and the extra hours proved overwhelming. I have never had the opportunity to speak with him again. As with many others, he went back into "the system," and I cannot contact him there because of privacy regulations. I cannot get an address, a phone number, or even a confirmation that he is alive or receiving services.

Sheila told me in a 2009 phone conversation that she thought Isaac's work experiences at PEP harmed his mental well-being. "There was too much pressure on him. Pressure at work," she observed. On top of too many hours, Sheila thought the newly-required, computer-based fee-for-service documentation of every fifteen minutes spent with each member pushed him over the edge. His off-site supervisor agreed. By the time Isaac left, he told me, "he couldn't stand feeling like he didn't know what he was doing on the computer, and he had very limited writing skills." In one interpretation, we could say that Isaac had stopped feeling that people saw him as a good person, and that he could contribute to the common good of PEP. Without this sense of moral agency, he began to lose his capacity for recovery.

Sheila also left PEP not long after Isaac. When she received a full Horizons scholarship to work on her master's degree in social work, Vera recruited her to work full-time at PEP instead. Sheila decided to stay because she had to send her own child to college that year, and she felt her job at PEP, as opposed to going back to school, put her in a better financial position at that moment. A few months after she started full-time work at PEP, though, Sheila also had a relapse after four years of stability.

During our January 2009 conversation, Sheila shared that her relapse lasted two years and was rooted in problems with her doctors and her medications:

> My doctor that was so great, you know? Well she just kind of freaked out. There were too many medications, and she just kept pushing them higher, but they weren't working. So then, I had to leave her and go through a bunch of idiot doctors, and I had *five* hospitalizations until I found a more empathic doctor.

Sheila also thought problems at PEP contributed to her relapse:

> That's why I left. I felt so much pressure to not take a day off and to do everything, and it was just too much. I had to protect myself, too, and I felt bad because Isaac and I both had to leave, but that was it. Vera just wanted too much. We were pushing ourselves too hard to do everything. You know, Vera can turn it on and do it all but it just wore me out. It wore us all out.

Isaac was never fired. Horizons let his sick leave run out, and then let him go. This enabled them to bypass the rules about accommodating workers in the Americans with Disabilities Act (1990). They did the same with Sheila.

When I asked where Isaac was in 2009, Sheila said he was worse.

I did a lot to help Isaac. We were really tight there for a while, but he has gotten to the point now where you can't even talk to him. He's not reachable. We decided we shouldn't talk for a while. We just looked at each other and said, "Oh, my God, we are both in hell right now, and we can't help each other right now." So we stopped talking. Isaac is doing really bad.

Around the same time, Vera told me that Isaac was in a "recovery home." I wondered if that was her new term for a nursing home. She gave me his number, but when I called, the number was no longer his.

I lost Isaac like I lost Maison. I may never see him again, and I miss him.

Sheila, on the other hand, seemed to be doing well. She worked part-time at a program facilitating peer services. She said much of her success could be attributed to the support of her family and the man she planned to marry (and did)—a very intelligent and kind man who was also a peer.

I also met Melanie, the peer Director of Recovery who had resigned, for lunch in Spring 2007. To my disappointment, she resisted discussing Horizons. Instead, she told me she missed being a therapist and administrative pressures and deadlines did not suit her. "I would rather work somewhere a little more low-key," she said softly, "where I think I can deliver what they are looking for, and not be disappointing people all the time."

Joel and Vera were the only people working at PEP when I visited in 2009. At this point, PEP had been moved to a new location, and the staff had been reduced to three. When I asked Joel how he survived as a peer provider, he shared his "most important skill: the ability to say no." Joel had attended college classes while working at PEP, so he had limited hours and never accepted extra hours without reasonable notice. Joel believed his most important job, as a peer provider, was to maintain his own mental health. If he did not feel well, he claimed, he could not help anyone else.

When Joel experienced depressive symptoms, he called his doctor, took a day off, and then returned to work. He needed the rest, he said, and then the return to work and his colleagues helped his symptoms subside.

In one email, Vera seemed wistful about all of the changes. "I miss Sheila and Isaac," she wrote in Spring 2009. The job and what took place may have been too much for them. They were great at it and born to do this job."

The Good Fight

Vera told me that despite all of the setbacks, she wanted to continue to "fight the good fight." In February 2009, we tramped through knee-high snow to visit Darcy, who, Vera said, was forty-two and had been living in a nursing home for ten years.

"The only reason that she is living there that I can figure out," Vera told me, "is that her mother doesn't want to have to worry about her. She's become childlike, but I think if she can learn to cook for herself, she can take care of her own place, and be her own payee."

Thanks to PEP's advocacy and action, Darcy would partake in a pilot program (later cancelled by mental health funding cuts) that charged her only 30 percent of her disability benefits for rent. She could spend the rest of her SSI check (probably around $450) on necessities. At the time, for a person living on SSI (currently $710/month), this was an incredible deal. Even though Americans are advised to only spend one third of their income on rent, users living on disability incomes easily spend most of their income on housing.

As we made our way to the nursing home, giant plumes of steam erupted from crystalline skyscrapers.

"We have a great set up at the hotel, don't you think?" Vera asked. That morning, I had attended PEP's weekly peer meeting at the new location—a single-room occupancy hotel upriver in an area known as the "psychiatric ghetto." PEP operated there on Thursday and Friday mornings, and at the Horizons Recovery Center on Saturday and Sunday (when Riverside was not open). PEP's staff offices moved to Horizons headquarters where the non-peer supervisor had more contact with peer staff.

Their focus was now on helping people transition out of nursing homes by providing them with an intimate network of peers in their new home at the hotel. The peers came to visit during their first week, brought them meals, and showed them the ropes of community life.

"It's the real peer support model, you know?" she said firmly. "No staff—just peers helping peers. They will bring Darcy her meals the first week and show her the ropes and make sure she isn't lonely or afraid. It will make the whole transition easier for her."

Using intimacy to foster moral agency, I would now say, was key to Vera's approaches, even if we could not name it at the time. Once inside the nursing home, Vera and I made our way into a windowless office where Darcy sat with her nurse. She reminded me of a china doll—cropped, silver hair and barely-lined porcelain skin from years inside. She stared intently at a spot on the table while Vera spent about twenty minutes advocating for her release.

After asking Vera questions about the place where Darcy would move, and how she would learn to cook and do her own laundry, the nurse agreed she was ready to leave. She left the room to "start the paperwork" and wished us a good day.

"Are you excited, Darcy?" Vera asked after the nurse left.

"When do I get my money?" Darcy mumbled.

"Oh!" Vera whooped. "You are excited about getting to be your own payee? Darcy has been living on thirty dollars per month for ten years, Neely," she said to me. "How do you think that feels?"

I nodded sympathetically at Darcy, but I really had no idea how that would feel. I thought my research stipend was awful, and I received about one thousand dollars per month. She was still not looking at us.

"We're going to get you your own money and your own apartment in a nice place. And the people from PEP will be there. And, hey!" she added, looking stern. "Where have you been? I haven't seen you at PEP in a couple of weeks!"

"It's been too cold," Darcy squeaked.

"Too cold?" Vera asked incredulously. "Too cold for recovery?"

"No," Darcy responded timidly. "They won't let us out. They said it's too cold, so we're locked in."

"Okay, okay. Well, when you're not in this nursing home anymore, no one can tell you that." Vera shot me a look that said—can you imagine, nursing homes locking in grown adults? Then she took Darcy's hands in her own and gave them a squeeze.

"Well," Vera said, "I am just saying this because we miss you, and we can't wait for you to move in."

"Really?" Darcy looked at me for the first time. I smiled and nodded encouragingly.

"Really," Vera promised.

A sweet smile crinkled Darcy's mouth.

Vera's program did not erase psychiatric disability or cure people. One person that PEP had helped to leave a nursing home, an administrator told me, even committed suicide two years later. This was very hard for Vera, the administrator added. But sitting there with Darcy, it was clear that something about the unconditional intimacy that Vera offered people—the touch, the smile, the empathy, the humanness—seemed an antidote to the toxic rejection that dominated most members' everyday lives.

Radical Hope

In his book about Chief Plenty Coups, the last chief of the Crow Nation, philosopher Jonathan Lear talks about "radical hope" in the face of "cultural devastation" (Lear 2006). While the situation of the Crow was very different and profoundly dire—they rapidly lost access to their homelands and traditional way of life—experiencing a serious mental illness in the United States is in some ways a similar experience. Lear's book describes the "cultural devastation" experienced by the Crow Nation when they lost their sense of what it meant to be a good person after the eradication of their nomadic, "courage-based" culture on the Great Plains. As people with serious mental illnesses enter treatment—and so often lose their relationships, jobs, and life goals—they are separated from their sense of how they might become recognized as good people and so live moral lives. Horizons members experienced cultural devastation when they could no longer work, and there was no cultural alternative to help them continue to lead a valued life. Work is the key to moral regard in mainstream US culture. Without work, the members no longer knew how to act in a way that earned the regard of others and enabled them to become moral agents. They could not access the intimate relationships they needed to learn how to thrive. Members struggled to develop their capacity to reimagine what it meant to be good and to lead a good life.

Lear argued that the Crow were ultimately saved by "radical hope," or an ability to imagine a future way of leading a good life even when a person or a society lacks the concepts with which to anticipate what this future will be. Chief Plenty Coups, for example, used the cultural tradition of sharing dreams (literally, a dream he had while sleeping) to convey a better future to his people, which ultimately enabled them to move forward. This capacity to dream, to imagine, and to become anew through a hope that illuminates a way forward through a new set of virtues in the company of intimate others is radical hope. Such hope—as Dr. Martin Luther King once proposed in his "I Have a Dream" speech—can be hewn only by dreamers from a mountain of despair.

In this book, we have walked with Vera as she enacted her own dream to usher profoundly dispossessed people toward some modicum of freedom and intimacy in recovery. We have journeyed with them to the edge of what is possible in the current model of recovery. Now it is time to employ a radical hope in imagining what is needed to complete the journey.

During my time with Vera I witnessed how she helped others plant seeds of radical hope. These seeds, in retrospect, were first made available by the initial proponents of recovery—the people in recovery, the family members, the caring professionals, the policymakers—all in search of a new way for their loved ones to heal from serious emotional distress. And this radical hope, I now know, can only continue to take root and blossom if people are willing to look beyond a person's economic value and recognize another human life. Addressing serious mental illness in the United States will never be cheap or convenient, but it must become an ethical imperative.

OVER THE EDGE | 7

"You have been the veterans of creative suffering. Continue to work with the faith that
unearned suffering is redemptive."

—*Martin Luther King Jr., August 28, 1963*

Of the more than 8.5 million individuals diagnosed with serious mental illnesses in the United States, one person out of twenty from the "extremely vulnerable group" receive *minimally adequate* mental health care each year (Wang, Demler, and Kessler 2002). Enter Horizons, embracing the new era of recovery. As an organization well positioned to take on the Sisyphean task of promoting recovery in the fragmented mental health system, Horizons seemed like a good place to test how a recovery-oriented philosophy might change care as usual in real time. This ethnography has examined how Horizons' efforts to become more recovery-oriented impacted the everyday lives of the members and staff who were required— often not by choice—to live by the rules, roles, and relationships prescribed for them. I have argued that mental health care reform efforts at Horizons, despite stated good intentions, continued to foreclose opportunities for members.

Recovery—as described by Horizons—was very difficult for members to achieve. In Horizons' interpretation of the recovery process, a person would take a "recovery journey" of three steps: to become rational, and then autonomous, and then hard working, and so prove themselves worthy of intimate connections with others. However, this branding of recovery sets a high bar for members who were profoundly stigmatized and alienated in a society in which they have long been thought of as "moral leeches" in the public imagination (Nussbaum 2006). To even consider a journey of recovery, this book has made plain, members needed strong, intimate, reciprocal, accountable relationships with caring others from the very beginning—relationships that most members had with no one. I have called the ability to cultivate this kind of intimacy moral agency. The concept of moral agency suggests that in order for people to become the kind of person they want to be in the world, they must act in a way that helps others recognize them as the person they hope to be and holds them accountable for it. The way that they are expected to act in order to be perceived as "good" must match up with the cultural expectations of the group that they are trying to join, and they will need resources that go beyond financial assistance to help replenish lost moral agency. This book has illustrated the many ways that members' experiences in mental health care had eroded their moral agency to a point where they needed more help restoring it than the mental health system offered them.

In practice, then, Horizons' "recovery journey" set members up to fail. Trapped in an ever-shifting landscape of poverty, crime, hunger, and physical and emotional pain that was somehow always different (a new shelter, a new alleyway, a new nursing home) and always the same (surrounded by "paid friends" and people suffering, facing victimization in the world "out there," few opportunities for gainful employment, medical insurance that required them to remain sick enough to afford their medications), the members I met struggled to survive, often alone. Despite the promise of the recovery journey at Horizons, the inadequacy of an imagined pharmaceutical cure for "broken brains," the strikingly stressful living conditions of members' lives, and their seemingly unrelenting isolation from mainstream US society persisted. While getting people back to work is a great idea, members needed care of a very different sort to address the demoralization, misrecognition, existential crises, and catastrophic conditions of everyday survival that affected them most. Radically different relationships, roles, and resources were needed to help people invigorate their ability to be recognized as moral agents, or a "good" community member accountable for their own actions in a way that made possible intimate connections. In sum, recovery is real, but people need to be supported in their recoveries in a fundamentally different way than Horizons put forth.

Horizons wanted members to learn to choose to recover. The idea that recovery can be achieved by choice, this book suggests, builds on US cultural values about what it means to be a good, valued citizen. To become such a person, a service user presumably needed only to make the right choices. They simply needed to take medications, to act with enlightened self-interest, and to work hard. The truth is that these are impossible choices when, with a few exceptions, people outside of the center did not see members as valuable adults worthy of relationship. They had profoundly eroded moral agency, and expecting people with diminished moral agency to even have access to choices much less the good support needed to make them only set people up to fail.

Logics of Care

Philosopher Annemarie Mol's (2008) critical ethnographic analysis of current diabetes treatment, *The Logic of Care*, sheds some light on how we might move forward. Mol argued that a health care system based on the "logic of choice" expected rational, autonomous patients to make health care decisions. This kind of health care, however, fuelled patients' desires for freedom by choice, and gave them the impression that they were in control of their bodies. As Mol (2008:83), who herself suffers from chronic diabetes, wisely stated: "active patients . . . have to be energetic as well as resigned about their own suffering. It is not to be underestimated, this huge emotional and practical effort. And yet it is likely to be better than the illusion that you might control the world. For dreams of control do not make you happy. They make you neurotic. And one way or the other, they end in disappointment."

Mol (2008) argues that instead of the logic of choice, we should use the "logic of care" for people with chronic illnesses like diabetes—and, I would add, perhaps some people with psychiatric disabilities. The logic of care, Mol claimed, acknowledges that: 1) patients cannot always make rational, autonomous choices; 2) they can benefit from others' knowledge about the pros and cons of the choices available to them; and 3) patients are often active even if they are sharing decision-making with clinicians or others. Mol expected that a health care system for diabetics guided by a logic of care would offer patients more time with care providers, emotional support, and opportunities to actively make adaptive choices with guidance, when requested, from clinicians. Instead of independent, free-choosing, self-made patients dictating their own care, care would be "shaped and reshaped depending on results"—results that mattered for the lived experience of that particular individual and the people with whom they had intimate relationships (Mol 2008:20). Treatment setbacks (relapse) would be unpleasant surprises without moral weight. People would be encouraged to focus on "living with disease, rather than 'normality' as a standard" (Mol 2008:31). In the context of psychiatric disability, Davidson and colleagues (2009:69) have similarly advocated for system reform that makes possible a "form of recovery that does not require cure or remission of symptoms but that allows for—and only really makes sense within the context of—continued disability."

The logic of care is also evident in recovery advocates' original ideas before they were absorbed by the mental health system and its preoccupation with producing productive citizens. "Recovery is a process, a way of life, and attitude, and a way of approaching the day's challenges. The need is to meet the challenge of the disability and to reestablish a new and valued sense of integrity and purpose within and beyond the limits of the disability," Ridgway and colleagues wrote (2002:5). The logic of care can also be seen in the local brand of recovery surfacing among advocates in Toronto, who collectively agreed that "living with" a situation through "coping" and "acceptance" was a more realistic goal than "'recovery from' in the sense of effecting a cure" (Mental Health "Recovery" Study Working Group 2009:19).

Advocate Deegan also presaged the importance of the logic of care in her discussion of an advertisement for depression medication picturing a mother and daughter joyously running up the stairs next to a crayoned note from the child stating: "I got my mommy back." Deegan (2002) wrote: "the power of such images and advertising . . . has become a cultural expectation of how all illness should end happily ever after. For those of us who have struggled for years . . . [this] storyline does not hold true. . . . Transformation rather than restoration becomes our path."

Mol's logic of care enacted in peer service settings may offer the principles and space recovery advocates need to bring their radical hope that recovery is possible for all to fruition. At the heart of Mol's ideas about using the logic of care is the recognition that people trying to live with chronic disabilities must partner with care providers and loved ones to flourish along the way. Another aspect is that one should accept that one has a disability, and ask that others allow one to live with one's disability rather than expecting one to be normal and earn one's moral worth in the same ways as others. Well-supported peer services that use the logic of care and focus on helping people build a sense of moral agency may offer the space, respect, encouragement, flexibility, and time service users need to give and receive such care.

The Potential of Peer Services

Psychosocial rehabilitation organizations with long-entrenched institutional cultures like Horizons have long been quagmires for reform (Estroff 1981; Floersch 2002; Jacobson 2004). Fresh social contexts in which to implement recovery initiatives are needed. The good news is that recovery advocates have been doggedly developing grassroots, innovative, peer-run alternatives to traditional treatment for years that attempt to offer users compassionate care, mutual respect, and empathic relationships (Chamberlin 1978; Corrigan 2006; Davidson, Rowe, and Tondora 1999; Hardiman and Segal 2003; Mead and Hilton 2003; Zinman, Harp, and Budd 1987). PEP was one such service (that was also ill-supported in terms of training, space, support for staff, competitive wages, and the list goes on), but it was not the only one. In fact, many peer services have emerged that are better equipped to promote recovery.

Even in the absence of standardized "best practices" for peer services, most peer models in use help participants feel more hopeful, deal with daily stressors, and improve their sense of empowerment and daily experiences of recovery (Corrigan 2006; Hodges, Hardiman, and Segal 2004; Segal, Silverman, and Temkin 1995; Swarbrick 2007). Studies suggest that well-trained peers are able to not only offer professional counsel and have similar effects on people as professionally-licensed social workers (Chinman et al. 2000), but they may also better understand what service users were going through, which has been termed "shared humanness" (Davidson et al. 1999; Mead and Hilton 2003; Schutt and Rogers 2009; West 2011). In some states, Medicaid is now reimbursing peer services. In my own state of Texas, non-profits like the Hogg Foundation are rolling out well-supported peer networks statewide.

Licensed peer care providers have been shown to be at least as effective as their professional counterparts in some care situations, such as working with homeless people with serious mental illnesses (Chinman et al. 2000). Currently peer-based care providers offer a range of services, including: promoting self-determination, personal responsibility, and health and wellness education; combatting stigma and hopelessness; and providing communication assistance between peers and care providers (e.g., psychiatrists) (Salzer, Schwenk, and Brusilovskiy, 2010). The peer-led, self-help, Wellness Recovery Action Program (WRAP) (Copeland 1997), for example, reduced psychiatric symptoms, increased hope, and improved participants' quality of life over time in a recent randomized clinical trial (Cook et al. 2012). Another peer-led intervention, Health and Recovery Program, for people diagnosed with a serious mental illness and a chronic medical illness, also improved health-related quality of life, physical activity, and people's willingness to take their medications (Druss et al. 2010).

In general, peer-led interventions have been successful, but more research is needed (Clay et al. 2005; Lloyd-Evans et al.

2014). Recent reviews call for further work in low-resource settings (for examples, see Fuhr et al. 2014 and Pitt et al. 2013), where lay health workers can help people learn local ways to manage mental health symptoms while connecting them with basic care (Balaji et al. 2012; Chatterjee et al. 2011). Lay health workers, such as peer providers, may help people find treatment more quickly, reduce stigma, encourage help-seeking, and protect and replenish a person's moral agency. Moreover, they likely can be introduced early on in the process of care, before the work of moral repair becomes more difficult, or a young person in crisis becomes a middle-aged person with twenty years behind them during which nothing seemed to happen.

Future research need not only ask whether or not peer services work, but also under what circumstances (Chinman et al. 2014). I would argue that peer services will be most effective in settings that work to respect, preserve, and enhance a person's moral agency. Interventions targeting one's capacity for moral agency could preserve and promote dignity and the social bases of self-respect, build on the potential of autobiographical power in mental health recovery, and cultivate viable communities in which people might live and thrive more seamlessly. Mental health care models that pay attention to the importance of moral agency and incorporate local peer care providers who understand the local culture show great promise for the future of mental health care.

Peer organizations that are outside of mainstream institutions help people develop capacities for self-determination, informed life-changing commitments, and increased social integration—the seeming goal of most recovery projects (Chamberlin, Rogers, and Ellison 1996; Corrigan et al. 2002; Hardiman and Segal 2003; Hopper 2007a; Ware et al. 2008). Two-way relationships between "peers" (peer providers and members) often are cited as a source of "family" for people who may be out of touch with their own—something we could see happening at PEP, as well (Lewis, Hopper and Healion 2012; Mental Health "Recovery" Study Working Group 2009). Peer-run organizations may also serve as a kind of civic association or "locus of citizenship" that connects users to other community organizations (Tanenbaum 2011). Such relationships may increase the civic activity of services users and decrease societal stigma by increasing contact (Davidson 2009; Hardiman and Segal 2003; Sayce 2000). These are all, I would argue, potential resources for restoring moral agency.

The Next Horizon

PEP was obviously not the ideal peer service model. Investigating peer programs that are legitimate examples of the possibilities of reform is critical to making sure that all peer services are not dismissed based on the evaluation of programs (like PEP) that are not state-of-the-art. This was not Vera's fault; she lacked the freedom and resources so many other peer service models are now trying to secure from the beginning.

One program that deserves more attention is Hands Across Long Island (HALI), which has recently been selected by the New York Office of Mental Health as a model with which to replace failing, traditional mental health care programs. HALI, which has been twenty years in the making, uses the "evidence-based" Personal Recovery-Oriented Services (PROS) protocol developed in partnership with the New York Office of Mental Health (NYOMH 2009) to provide recovery-oriented, Medicaid-reimbursable services. These services include a drop-in center, peer-run clinical services (including a peer therapist, peer nurse, and peer psychiatrist), an in-house HALI University educational program, a dual-diagnosis program, and an advocacy program. In 2011, I had the opportunity to conduct nine months of ethnographic fieldwork at one of HALI's new locations in New York and see their model in action, as well as to collaborate with anthropologist Sara Lewis, who had conducted a formal, ten-month ethnography of the original HALI in partnership with Kim Hopper and Ellen Healion, the director (Lewis, Hopper, and Healion 2012).

Why does HALI thrive while PEP did not? While both served large populations—HALI serves 3,500 people each year, as a stand-alone, grassroots peer organization, HALI lacked Horizons' institutional legacy of traditional mental health care. HALI even has the nation's first peer-run mental health clinic, which means that the prescribing mental health care provider is a peer that values peer input. HALI's peer environment valued people and asked them to be responsible for each other and hold each accountable from the beginning of their service use, rather than expecting people to self-actualize on their own (Lewis, Hopper, and Healion 2012). And unlike PEP, HALI was never subjected to the non-peer supervision that can debilitate the efficacy of peer programs (Mowbray, Robinson, and Holter 2002). HALI's staff and participants did not have to prove themselves to skeptics like Riverside staff and Horizons administrators who kept PEP on a short leash. They were not competing for members or trying to establish rules alongside a philosophically incompatible program as with PEP and Riverside.

Innovations in peer services may also combine well with other proposed new directions in care that promote recovery. While it remains controversial, some argue that early intervention may limit disability for young people after they are first diagnosed with a psychotic disorder, much like treating cancer as early as possible for a better outcome (McGorry 2011). In this model, youth who are connected to treatment quickly have less time to burn bridges with family, friends, and employers and seem to have less disability over time (Lloyd-Evans et al. 2011; Marshall et al. 2005). What if young people were offered a peer-led intervention as soon as they had a psychotic break that kept them from feeling alienated, helped preserve their moral agency, and inspired them to continue to seek care? We need some young peers who are doing well to lead such an initiative, the research to back it up, and the funding to do it. The National Mental Health Consumers' Self-Help Clearinghouse is currently leading this conversation.

Another useful peer-led technique may be one developed by the Hearing Voices Network, now Intervoice (*www.intervoice.org*), which teaches people how to dialogue with their "voices" in order to better understand and control them in supportive groups of people who hear voices (Escher, Hage, and Romme 1998; Romme 2000; Romme and Escher 1989; Romme et al., 2009). In these groups, people who hear voices meet other people who are not necessarily in psychiatric treatment and who share similar experiences. Most of these groups are community-based and free to attend. Such interventions may help preserve or replenish moral agency as people bond over shared experiences and resist troubling symptoms that often harm one's relationships with others. We will ultimately need a strong evidence base to secure more public support for these innovations in care.

~ • ~

HAVING READ THIS BOOK, you may be tempted to say, "recovery does not work"; or, "mad people in the United States are too disabled to recover." Such a conclusion is premature and incorrect. We need different venues, and different roles, rules, and relationships, for recovery principles to stand a chance. Peer services show promise for informing how the logic of care may be incorporated into symptom management for people with psychiatric disabilities, and help users replenish their moral agency. Early interventions show promise for an upstream disruption of the erosion of moral agency that mental health services often perpetuate. Peer-led early interventions may be ideal. As people in recovery around the globe find and share novel, locally meaningful ways to heal, we can build an evidence-base for services that help people restore a diminished sense of moral agency—and protect it from erosion in the first place. In this way—together—as so many have hoped, we may finally render the "revolving-door, chronic mental patient" a haunting and regrettable relic of our misguided past.

APPENDIX

Comparison of Traditional and Recovery-as-Advocated Care

Principles	Care as Usual (Traditional)	Recovery-as-Advocated Model*
Goals	*Rehabilitation:* stabilize illness, reduce negative impacts of illness, avoid rehospitalization	*Recovery:* community reintegration; meaningful life; minimize negative impacts of "traditional" treatment
Assumptions	Services reduce "impairments, dysfunctions, disabilities, and disadvantages"	Anyone can achieve recovery with hope, empowerment, and peer support
Treatment Locales	Psychiatric hospitals, nursing homes, community-based centers	Added option of peer-run programs, drop-in centers, and respite centers
Treatment Relationship	*Case manager:* educated, licensed clinical directs client; physical, narrative, and emotional boundaries limit reciprocity	*Peer Provider:* experienced former mental health service user as adviser; collaborative decision-making; reciprocity encouraged
Key Terminology	Compliant, stable, adherent, non-rehospitalized	Freedom, empowerment, hope, autonomy, self-determination, social reintegration, anti-coercion, self-advocacy

Medications	Prescribe and comply; involuntary or forced treatment when necessary; coercion is for client's own good	Educate and support; avoid involuntary treatment and coercion; use "advance directives" and shared decision-making
Money Management	Guardian/payee relationship	Learn independence by trial and error
Personal Choice	*Paternalistic caretaking:* users need help to make the right choices when they are "sick"	*Self-determination:* learn personal responsibility by making their own choices even if they try and fail
Employment	Some people can't work due to their psychiatric disability and need government disability benefits to survive	Anyone can work with proper support; no one should be expected to live on meager disability benefits
Housing	Nursing homes and other protected environments	Affordable and safe housing in the least restrictive setting

* Recovery-as-advocated is not the model Horizons used, but the model originally put forth by advocates.

NOTES

CHAPTER 1

1. Horizons is a pseudonym, used at their request. However, they do have a copy of my preliminary findings, and I have also discussed my findings in conversations with some of the staff, administrators, and members.
2. Peer Empowerment Program and PEP are also both pseudonyms.

CHAPTER 2

1. Members receiving SSI who then found employment were subject to "earnings disregard" rules. A person who wanted to maintain SSI (and their health insurance) could not have a monthly income over $988.50, meaning they could only work at minimum wage for about 127 hours each month (160 is considered to be "full-time") before they lost their benefits, including the disability income check, Medicaid, special reduced transportation fares (80 cents per ride instead of two dollars in 2009), and food stamps (alone worth $167 per month). Thus, members on needs-based SSI lost all of their benefits if they tried to work full time.
2. Clients and staff used the term *mouthing meds* to describe what people did when they held administered medications in their mouths rather than swallowing them until they found a way to spit out the medications without being detected.
3. Norm is a character from a hit US TV show called *Cheers* that aired from 1982 to 1993.
4. Working hard, however, at least according to the literature, was not always the best prescription for mental health. Social and economic mobility in America, one physician lamented, caused people to have "more groundless hopes, and more painful struggles to obtain that which is beyond reach, or to effect that which is impossible" (Jarvis 1852). Historian Alexis De Tocqueville (2000) similarly observed that Americans, despite being the "freest and most enlightened" were "almost sad, even in their pleasures," for they were "forever brooding over advantages they [did] not possess."

CHAPTER 3

1. Lithium and Depakote are used to treat mood swings.
2. Maison is referring here to a newer atypical antipsychotic medication, clozapine, for which people have to take a blood test once each week for the first six months and then every two weeks indefinitely thereafter. This medicine affects the white blood cell count and can lead to death if not monitored.
3. I only attended this group once, but after that decided I did not want to accidentally interrupt any male bonding.
4. The vast majority of members were on medications, but I confirmed that at least six members were not on medications at any point during my study.
5. Later, a reader of this text (and long-time medication user) told me she thought "numbed out" would be a better description of what medicated members likely felt after taking anti-anxiety medications.
6. I met at least eight members who, for at least six weeks of their time at the center, used drugs and alcohol to "self-medicate" rather than taking psychiatric medication.
7. While many people in various programs who were taking psychiatric drugs told me that they faced criticism from the Narcotics Anonymous and Alcoholics Anonymous communities for doing so or used this perhaps as an explanation for why they did not attend these meetings, a restriction against medication is not in the official rules of these organizations.

CHAPTER 4

1. At this point in American history, "ground zero" was a very loaded term used to refer to the zone of culture clash and discontent that the Ground Zero of 9/11 had come to represent.
2. For more, see Brodwin's (2012) excellent ethnography of "everyday ethics" in community psychiatry—a look at the difficult decisions frontline ACT case managers must make every day.
3. For historian Alexis de Tocqueville (2000 [1840]) American "enlightened" self-interest contrasted with the European model of self-serving, aristocratic self-interest. The right to act in accordance with one's own self-interests, economist Adam Smith (1904 [1776] might argue, was due to the "invisible hand" guiding actors in capitalist societies. Smith's "invisible hand" leads a rational actor to pursue his own interests in an "enlightened" way that promotes the interests of many even though this is often not the direct intention of the actor.

CHAPTER 6

1. In a Winter 2009 email, a Horizons administrator wrote: "Peer staff do, indeed, go through New Staff Orientation like everyone else who is employed at Horizons. You are right, there was and is no special module on non-violent crisis intervention as part of the package. . . . We also offer a regular training (every six months or so) called Crisis Management and Response which incorporates elements of aggression management, verbal de-escalation, etc.

REFERENCES

Abu-Lughod, Lila
  1986   *Veiled Sentiments: Honor and Poetry in a Bedouin Society.* Berkeley: University of California Press.
ADA, Americans with Disabilities Act of 1990
  1990   Pub. L. No. 101-336, 104 Stat. 328
Andreasen, Nancy C.
  1984   *The Broken Brain: The Biological Revolution in Psychiatry.* New York: Harper and Row.
Angell, Beth
  2003   Contexts of Social Relationship Development Among Assertive Community Treatment Clients. *Mental Health Services Research* 5(1):13–25.
  2006   Measuring Strategies Used by Mental Health Providers to Increase Medication Adherence. *Journal of Behavioral Health and Services Research* 33(1):53–72.
Angell, Beth, and Colleen Mahoney
  2007   Reconceptualizing the Case Management Relationship in Intensive Treatment: A Study of Staff Perceptions and Experiences. *Administration and Policy in Mental Health and Mental Health Services Resesarch* 34(2):172–88.
Angell, Beth, Colleen Mahoney, and Noriko I. Martinez
  2006   Promoting Adherence in Assertive Community Treatment. *Social Service Review* 80(3):485–526.
Anthony, William A.
  1993   Recovery From Mental Illness: The Guiding Vision of the Mental Health Service System in the 1990s. *Psychosocial Rehabilitation Journal* 16(4):11–23.
  2000   A Recovery-Oriented Service System: Setting Some System Level Standards. *Psychiatric Rehabilitation Journal* 24(2):159–68.
APA, American Psychiatric Association
  2000   *Diagnostic and Statistical Manual of Mental Disorders: DSM-IV-TR.* Washington, DC: American Psychiatric Association.
  2004   Practice Guidelines for the Treatment of Patients with Schizophrenia. *American Journal of Psychiatry* 161:1–56.
Balaji, Madhumitha, Sudipto Chatterjee, Mirja Koschorke, Thara Rangaswamy, Animish
Chavan, Hamid Dabholkar, Lilly Dakshin, Pratheesh Kumar, Sujit John,
and Graham Thornicroft
  2012   The Development of a Lay Health Worker Delivered Collaborative Community Based Intervention for People with Schizophrenia in India. *BMC Health Services Research* 12(1):42.

Baron, Richard C.

1995   Establishing Employment Services as a Priority for Persons with Long-Term Mental Illness. *American Rehabilitation* 21(1):32–35.

Bassman, Ronald

2001   Overcoming the Impossible: My Journey Through Schizophrenia. *Psychology Today* (Jan/Feb):35–40.

Beard, John H., Rudyard N. Propst, and Thomas J. Malamud

1982   The Fountain House Model of Psychosocial Rehabilitation. *Psychosocial Rehabilitation Journal* 5(1):47–53.

Beers, Clifford W.

1960   [1908] *A Mind that Found Itself: An Autobiography*. New York: Doubleday.

Bell, Morris D., and Paul H. Lysaker

1997   Clinical Benefits of Paid Work Activity in Schizophrenia: 1-Year Followup. *Schizophrenia Bulletin* 23(2):317–28.

Bellack, Alan S., and Carlo C. DiClemente

1999   Treating Substance Abuse Among Patients with Schizophrenia. *Psychiatric Services* 50(1):75–80.

Bellah, Robert N., Richard Madsen, William M. Sullivan, Ann Swidler, and Steven M. Tipton

1996   *Habits of the Heart: Individualism and Commitment in American Life*. Berkeley: University of California Press.

Blacksher, Erika

2002   On Being Poor and Feeling Poor: Low Socioeconomic Status and the Moral Self. *Theoretical Medicine and Bioethics* 23(6): 455–70.

Bleuler, Eugen

1911   Dementia Praecox Oder die Gruppe der Schizophrenien. *In Hanbuch der Psychiatrie*. G. Aschaffenburg, ed. Leipzig, Germany: Deuticke.

Boykin, Cherie D.

1997   The Consumer Provider as Role Model. In *Consumers as Providers in Psychiatric Rehabilitation*. C. T. Mowbray, D. P. Moxley, C. A. Jasper, L. L. Howell, eds. Pp. 374–86. Columbia, MD: International Association of Psychosocial Rehabilitation Services.

Brock, Dan

1993   Quality of Life measures in Health Care and Medical Ethics. In *The Quality of Life*. M. C. Nussbaum and A. Sen, eds. Pp. 95–132. Oxford: Clarendon Press.

Brodwin, Paul

2008   The Coproduction of Moral Discourse in US Community Psychiatry. *Medical Anthropology Quarterly* 22(2):127–47.

2012   *Everyday Ethics: Voices from the Front Line of Community Psychiatry*. Berkeley: University of California Press.

Broussard, Beth, S. M. Goulding, C. L. Talley, and M. T. Compton

2010   Beliefs About Causes of Schizophrenia Among Urban African American Community Members. *Psychiatric Quarterly* 81(4):349–62.

Buchanan, David R.

2008   Autonomy, Paternalism, and Justice: Ethical Priorities in Public Health. *American Journal of Public Health* 98(1):15–21.

Buunk, Bram, and Aukje Nauta
: 2000   Why Intraindividual Needs are Not Enough: Human Motivation is Primarily Social. *Psychological Inquiry* 11(4):279–83.

Calabrese, Joseph D., and Patrick W. Corrigan
: 2005   Beyond Dementia Praecox: Findings from Long-Term Follow-Up Studies of Schizophrenia. In *Recovery in Mental Illness: Broadening our Understanding of Wellness*. R. O. Ralph and P. W. Corrigan, eds. Pp. 63–84. Washington, DC: American Psychological Association.

Caldwell, Anne E.
: 1978   History of Psychopharmacology. In *Principles of Psychopharmacology*. W. G. Clark and J. D. Giudice, eds. Pp. 9–40. New York: Academic.

Carling, Paul J.
: 1995   *Building Support Systems for People with Psychiatric Disabilities*. New York: Guilford Press.

Casey, Daniel E.
: 1999   Tardive Dyskinesia and Atypical Antipsychotic Drugs. *Schizophrenia Research* 35(Supplement 1):S61–66.

Chamberlin, Judi
: 1978   *On Our Own: Patient-Controlled Alternatives to the Mental Health System*. New York: McGraw-Hill.
: 1990   The Ex-Patients' Movement: Where We've Been and Where We're Going. *The Journal of Mind and Behavior* 11(3):323–36.

Chamberlin, Judi, E. Sally Rogers, and Marsha L. Ellison
: 1996   Self-help Programs: A Description of Their Characteristics and Their Members. *Psychiatric Rehabilitation Journal* 19(3):33–42.

Chatterjee, Sudipto, Leese Morven, Mirja Koschorke, Paul McCrone, Smita Naik, Sujit John, Hamid Dabholkar, Kimberley Goldsmith, Madhumita Balaji, and Mathew Varghese
: 2011   Collaborative Community Based Care for People and Their Families Living with Schizophrenia in India: Protocol for a Randomised Controlled Trial. *Trials* 12(1):12.

Chinman, Matthew, Robert Rosenheck, Julie Lam, and Larry Davidson
: 2000   Comparing Consumer and Nonconsumer Provided Case Management Services for Homeless Persons with Serious Mental Illness. *Journal of Nervous and Mental Disease* 188(7):446–53.

Chinman, Matthew, Preethy George, Richard H. Dougherty, Allen S. Daniels, Sushmita Shoma Ghose, Anita Swift, and Miriam E. Delphin-Rittmon
: 2014   Peer Support Services for Individuals with Serious Mental Illnesses: Assessing the Evidence. *Psychiatric Services* 65(4):429.

Choe, Jeanne Y., Linda A. Teplin, and Karen M. Abram
: 2008   Perpetration of Violence, Violent Victimization, and Severe Mental Illness: Balancing Public Health Concerns. *Psychiatric Services* 59(2):153–64.

Christensen, Richard C.
: 1997   Ethical Issues in Community Mental Health: Cases and Conflicts. *Community Mental Health Journal* 33(1):5–11.

Clay, Sally, Bonnie Schell, Patrick W. Corrigan, and Ruth O. Ralph
  2005   *On Our Own, Together: Peer Programs for People with Mental Illness.* Nashville, TN: Vanderbilt University Press.
Cohen, Mikal, B. Cohen, P. Nemec, M. Farkas, and R. Forbess
  1988   *Training Technology: Case Management.* Boston: Boston University Center for Psychiatric Rehabilitation.
Cohen, Oryx
  2001   *Psychiatric Survivor Oral Histories: Implications for Contemporary Mental Health Policy.* Capstone Report. Amherst, MA: Center for Public Policy and Administration, University of Massachusetts-Amherst.
Cook, Judith A.
  2006   Employment Barriers for Persons with Psychiatric Disabilities: A Report for the President's New Freedom Commission. *Psychiatric Services* 57:1391–405.
Cook, J. A., M. E. Copeland, J. A. Jonikas, M. M. Hamilton, L. A. Razzano, D. D. Grey, C. B. Floyd, W. B. Hudson, R. T. Macfarlane, and T. M. Carter
  2012   Results of a Randomized Controlled Trial of Mental Illness Self-Management using Wellness Recovery Action Planning. *Schizophrenia Bulletin* 38(4):881–91.
Copeland, Mary Ellen
  1997   *Wellness Recovery Action Plan.* Dummerston, VT: Peach Press.
  2008   *WRAP: Wellness Recovery Action Plan: WRAPPIn' Virginia in Recovery.* Richmond, VA: Virginia Department of Mental Health and Substance Abuse Services.
Corrigan, Patrick W.
  2006   Impact of Consumer-Operated Services on Empowerment and Recovery of People with Psychiatric Disabilities. *Psychiatric Services* 57(10):1493–96.
Corrigan, Patrick W., Joseph Calabrese, Sarah Diwan, Cornelius Keogh, Lorraine Keck, and Carol Mussey
  2002   Some Recovery Processes in Mutual-Help Groups for Persons with Mental Illness; I: Qualitative Analysis of Program Materials and Testimonies. *Community Mental Health Journal* 38(4):287–302.
CPR, Center for Psychiatric Rehabilitation
  1997   *Reasonable Accommodations: What is Psychiatric Disability and Mental Illness?*, Boston, MA: Boston University.
Crisp, Roger, and Brad Hooker, eds.
  2000   *Well-Being and Morality.* Oxford: Clarendon Press.
Crowley, Kathleen
  1996   What is Possible in Psychiatry: Five Psychiatric Steps that Mattered. *Psychiatric Rehabilitation Journal* 19(4):85–87.
Currier, Glenn W.
  2000   Datapoints: Psychiatric Bed Reductions and Mortality among Persons With Mental Disorders. *Psychiatric Services* 51(7):851.
Davidson, Larry, M. Chinman, B. Kloos, R. Weingarten, D. Stayner, and J. K. Tebes
  1999   Peer Support among Individuals with Severe Mental Illness: A Review of the Evidence. *Clinical Psychology: Science and Practice* 6:165–87.
Davidson, Larry, and Thomas H. McGlashan
  1997   The Varied Outcomes of Schizophrenia. *Canadian Journal of Psychiatry* 42(1):34–43.

Davidson, Larry, Michael Rowe, Janis Tondora, Maria J. O'Connell, and
Martha Staeheli Lawless
   2008   *A Practical Guide to Recovery-Oriented Practice: Tools for Transforming Mental Health
          Care.* Oxford: Oxford University Press.
Davis, Simon
   2002   Autonomy versus Coercion: Reconciling Competing Perspectives in Community
          Mental Health. *Community Mental Health Journal* 38(3):239–50.
Deegan, Gene
   2003   Discovering Recovery. *Psychiatric Rehabilitation Journal* 26(4):368–76.
Deegan, Patricia E.
   1988   Recovery: The Lived Experience of Rehabilitation. *Psychosocial Rehabilitation
          Journal* 11(4):11–19.
   1993   Recovering Our Sense of Value After Being Labeled Mentally Ill. *Journal of
          Psychosocial Nursing & Mental Health Services* 31(4):7–11.
   1996   Recovery and the Conspiracy of Hope. Sixth Annual Mental Health Services
          Conference of Australia and New Zealand, 1996.
   2002   Recovery as a Self-Directed Process of Healing and Transformation. *Occupational
          Therapy in Mental Health* 17(3/4):5–21.
Deegan, Patricia E., and Robert E. Drake
   2006   Shared Decision Making and Medication Management in the Recovery Process.
          Psychiatric Services 57(11):1636–39.
DeSisto, M. Jane, C. M. Harding, R. V. McCormick, T. Ashikaga, and G. W. Brooks
   1995   The Maine and Vermont Three-Decade Studies of Serious Mental Illness. *British
          Journal of Psychiatry* 167(3):331–42.
Desjarlais, Robert
   1996   The Office of Reason: On the Politics of Language and Agency in a Shelter for "The
          Homeless Mentally Ill." *American Ethnologist* 23(4):880–900.
DHHS, Department of Health and Human Services
   2003a *New Freedom Commission on Mental Health: Report of the Subcommittee on
          Consumer Issues: Shifting to a Recovery-Based Continuum of Care.* DHHA Pub No.
          SMW-03-3832: Rockville, MD: Author.
   2003b *New Freedom Commission on Mental Health: Achieving the Promise: Transforming
          Mental Health Care in America.* DHHA Pub No. SMW-03-3832: Rockville, MD:
          Author.
   2009   *The 2009 HHS Poverty Guidelines: One Version of the [US] Federal Poverty Measure.*
          Rockville, MD: Author.
Ditton, Paula M.
   1999   *Mental Health and Treatment of Inmates and Probationers.* Washington, DC: US
          Department of Justice.
Dixon, Lisa, Nancy Krauss, and Anthony Lehman
   1994   Consumers as Service Providers: The Promise and Challenge. *Community Mental
          Health Journal* 30(6):615–25.
Douglass, Frederick
   1992   Self-Made Men. In *The Frederick Douglass Papers.* J. W. Blassingame and J. R.
          McKivigan, eds. Pp. 545—575. Series One: Speeches, Debates, and Interviews,
          Vol. 4: 1881–1895. New Haven: Yale University Press.

Druss, Benjamin G., S. A. von Esenwein, M. T. Compton, K. J. Rask, L. Zhao, and R. M. Parker

    2010   The Health and Recovery Peer (HARP) Program: A Peer-Led Intervention to Improve Medical Self-Management for Persons with Serious Mental Illness. *Schizophrenia Research* 118(1):264–70.

Dworkin, Gerald

    1988   *The Theory and Practice of Autonomy*. Cambridge, England: Cambridge University Press.

Escher, Sandra, Patsy Hage, and Marius Romme

    1998   Maastricht Interview with a Voice-Hearer. In *Understanding Voices: Coping with Auditory Hallucinations and Confusing Realities*. M. Romme, ed. P. 57. Gloucester: Handsell Publishing.

Estroff, Sue E.

    1981   *Making It Crazy: An Ethnography of Psychiatric Clients in an American Community*. Los Angeles: University of California Press.

    2004   Subject/Subjectivities in Dispute: The Poetics, Politics, and Performance of First-Person Narratives of People with Schizophrenia. In *Schizophrenia, Culture, and Subjectivity: The Edge of Experience*. J. H. Jenkins and R. J. Barrett, eds. Pp. 282–302. Cambridge Studies in Medical Anthropology, Vol. 11. Cambridge: Cambridge University Press.

Farina, Amerigo, Donald Gilha, Louis Boudreau, Jon Allen, and Mark Sherman

    1971   Mental Illness and the Impact of Believing Others Know about It. *Journal of Abnormal Psychology* 77(1):1–5.

Farkas, M., C. Gagne, W. Anthony, and J. Chamberlin

    2005   Implementing Recovery Oriented Evidence Based Programs: Identifying the Critical Dimensions. *Community Mental Health Journal* 41(2):141–58.

Farmer, Paul

    2003   *Pathologies of Power: Health, Human Rights, and the New War on the Poor*. Volume 4. Berkeley: University of California Press.

Fekete, David J.

    2004   How I Quit Being a "Mental Patient" and Became a Whole Person with a Neuro-Chemical Imbalance: Conceptual and Functional Recovery from a Psychotic Episode. *Psychiatric Rehabilitation Journal* 28(2):189–94.

Fisher, Daniel B.

    1993   Towards a Positive Culture of Healing. In *The DMH Core Curriculum: Consumer Empowerment and Recovery, Part U*. Boston: Commonwealth of Massachusetts Department of Mental Health.

    1994   Hope, Humanity, and Voice in Recovery from Psychiatric Disability. *Journal of the California Alliance for the Mentally Ill* 5(3):7–11.

Fisher, Daniel B., and Judi Chamberlin

    2004   *Consumer-Directed Transformation to a Recovery-Based Mental Health System*. Boston, MA: National Empowerment Center.

Floersch, Jerry

    2002   *Meds, Money, and Manners*. New York: Columbia University Press.

Foley, Henry A.
1975 *Community Mental Health Legislation: The Formative Process.* Lexington, MA: Lexington Books.

Forbush, Bliss
1971 *The Sheppard & Enoch Pratt Hospital, 1853–1970: A History.* Philadelphia: Lippincott.

Foucault, Michel
1965 *Madness and Civilization: A History of Insanity in the Age of Reason.* New York: Random House, Inc.

Frese, Frederick
1998 Advocacy, Recovery, and the Challenges of Consumerism for Schizophrenia. *Psychiatric Clinics of North America* 21(1):233–49.

Frese, Frederick, Jonathan Stanley, Ken Kress, and Suzanne Vogel-Scibilia
2001 Integrating Evidence-Based Practices and the Recovery Model. *Psychiatric Services* 52(11):1462–69.

Fuhr, Daniela C., Tatiana T. Salisbury, Mary J. De Silva, Najia Atif, Nadja van Ginneken, Atif Rahman, and Vikram Patel
2014 Effectiveness of Peer-Delivered Interventions for Severe Mental Illness and Depression on Clinical and Psychosocial Outcomes: A Systematic Review and Meta-Analysis. *Social Psychiatry and Psychiatric Epidemiology.* Epub ahead of print 2014 Mar 17. Accessed May 8, 2014.

Gamwell, Lynn, and Nancy Tomes
1995 *Madness in America: Cultural and Medical Prescriptions of Mental Illness before 1914.* Ithaca, NY: Cornell University Press.

Garcia, Angela
2010 *The Pastoral Clinic: Addiction and Dispossession Along the Rio Grande.* Los Angeles: University of California Press.

Geddes, J., N. Freemantle, P. Harison, and P. Bebbington
2000 Atypical Antipsychotics in the Treatment of Schizophrenia: Systematic Overview and Meta-Regression Analysis. *British Medical Journal* 321(7273):1371–76.

Gioia, Deborah, and John S. Brekke
2003 Use of the Americans with Disabilities Act by Young Adults with Schizophrenia. *Psychiatric Services* 54(3):302–4.

Glass, Ira
1998 102: Road Trip! *This American Life* (radio show). Chicago: Chicago Public Media. *www.thisamericanlife.org/radio-archives/episode/102/road-trip.*

Goffman, Erving
1961 *Asylums: Essays on the Social Situation of Mental Patients and Other Inmates.* Aldine: Aldine Publishing Company.

Goldman, Howard H., Neal H. Adams, and Carl A. Taube
1983 Deinstitutionalization: The Data Demythologized. *Hospital and Community Psychiatry* 34(2):129–34.

Good, Mary-Jo DelVecchio
2001 The Biotechnical Embrace. *Culture, Medicine and Psychiatry.* 25(4):395–410.

Granger, Barbara

2000   The Role of Psychiatric Practitioners in Assisting People in Understanding How to Best Assert Their ADA Rights and Arrange Job Accommodations. *Psychiatric Rehabilitation Journal* 23(3):215–23.

Greenberg, Greg A., and Robert A. Rosenheck

2008   Jail Incarceration, Homelessness, and Mental Health: A National Study. *Psychiatric Services* 59(2):170–77.

Griffith, James L.

2010   *Religion that Heals, Religion that Harms: A Guide for Clinical Practice.* New York: The Guilford Press.

Grob, Gerald N.

1994   *The Mad Among Us: A History of the Care of America's Mentally Ill.* New York: Free Press.

Gronfein, William

1985   Incentives and Intentions in Mental Health Policy: A Comparison of the Medicaid and Community Mental Health Programs. *Journal of Health and Social Behavior* 26(3):192–206.

Hardiman, Eric R., and Steven P. Segal

2003   Community Membership and Social Networks in Mental Health Self Help Agencies. *Psychiatric Rehabilitation Journal* 27(1):25–33.

Harding, Courtenay M., Joseph Zubin, and John S. Strauss

1987   Chronicity in Schizophrenia: Fact, Partial Fact, or Artifact? *Schizophrenia Bulletin* 38(5):477–86.

Harwood, Henrick

2000   *The Economic Cost of Mental Illness.* Rockville, MD: National Institute for Mental Health.

Hawthorne, William B., D. P. Folsom, D. H. Sommerfeld, N. M. Lanouette, M. Lewis, G. A. Aarons, R. M. Conklin, E. Solorzano, L. A. Lindamer, and D. V. Jeste

2012   Incarceration among Adults Who Are in the Public Mental Health System: Rates, Risk Factors, and Short-Term Outcomes. *Psychiatric Services* 63(1):26–32.

Henderson, Holly

2004   From Depths of Despair to Heights of Recovery. *Psychiatric Rehabilitation Journal* 28(1):83–87.

Hodges, John Q., Eric R. Hardiman, and Steven P. Segal

2004   Hope Among Members of Mental Health Self-Help Agencies: A Descriptive Analysis. *Social Work in Mental Health* 2(1):1–16.

Hopper, Kim

2003   *Reckoning with Homelessness.* Ithaca, NY: Cornell University Press.

2007a Rethinking Social Recovery in Schizophrenia: What a Capabilities Approach Might Offer. *Social Science & Medicine* 65(5):868–79.

2007b *Recovery from Schizophrenia: An International Perspective: A Report from the WHO Collaborative Project, the International Study of Schizophrenia.* New York: Oxford University Press.

Hopper, Kim, J. Jost, T. Hay, S. Welber, and G. Haugland

1997   Homelessness, Severe Mental Illness, and the Institutional Circuit. *Psychiatric Services* 48(5):659–65.

Jacobson, Nora, and Laurie Curtis
  2000   Recovery as a Policy in Mental Health Services: Strategies Emerging from the
          States. *Psychiatric Rehabilitation Journal* 23(4):333–41.
Jacobson, Nora, Vanessa Oliver, and Andrew Koch
  2009   An Urban Geography of Dignity. *Health & Place* 15(3):725–31.
Jacobson, Nora
  2004   *In Recovery: The Making of Mental Health Policy.* Nashville: Vanderbilt University
          Press.
Jacobson, Nora, and Dianne Greenley
  2001   What Is Recovery? A Conceptual Model and Explication. *Psychiatric Services*
          52(4):482–85.
James, Doris J., and Lauren E. Glaze
  2006   *Mental Health Problems of Prison and Jail Inmates.* Washington, DC: US
          Department of Justice, Bureau of Justice Statistics.
Jarvis, Edward
  1852   On the Supposed Increase of Insanity. *American Journal of Psychiatry* 8:333–64.
Jenkins, Janis H.
  2010   Psychopharmaceutical Self and Imaginary in the Social Field of Psychiatric
          Treatment. In *Pharmaceutical Self: The Global Shaping of Experience in an Age of
          Psychopharmacology.* J. H. Jenkins, ed. Santa Fe: School for Advanced Research
          Press.
Jenkins, Janis H., and Elizabeth A. Carpenter-Song
  2008   Stigma Despite Recovery: Strategies for Living in the Aftermath of Psychosis.
          Medical Anthropology Quarterly 22(4):381–409.
Jenkins, Janis H., Milton E. Strauss, Elizabeth A. Carpenter, Dawn Miller, Jerry Floersch,
and Martha Sajatovic
  2005   Subjective Experience of Recovery from Schizophrenia-Related Disorders and
          Atypical Antipsychotics. *International Journal of Social Psychiatry* 51(3):211–27.
Jervis, E.
  1852   Insanity among the Coloured Population of the Free States. *The American Journal of
          Insanity* 8(4):331–61.
Jeste, Dilip V., J. P. Lacro, A. Bailey, and E. Rockwell
  1999   Lower Incidence of Tardive Dyskinesia with Risperidone Compared with
          Haloperidol in Older Patients. *Journal of the American Geriatrics Society* 47(6):716–
          19.
Jimenez, Mary Ann
  1987   *Changing Faces of Madness: Early American Attitudes and the Treatment of the Insane.*
          Hanover, NH: Brandeis University Press.
Kane, John M., and Thomas H. McGlashan
  1995   Treatment of Schizophrenia. *Lancet* 346(8978):820–25.
Kerouac, Jack
  2002   [1957] *On the Road.* New York: Penguin Classics.
Kikkert, Martijn J., Aart H. Schene, Maarten W. J. Koeter, Debbie Robson, Anja Born,
Hedda Helm, Michela Nose, Glaudia Goss, Graham Thornicroft, and Richard J. Gray
  2006   Medication Adherence in Schizophrenia: Exploring Patients', Carers' and
          Professionals' Views. *Schizophrenia Bulletin* 32(4):786–94.

Kirmayer, Laurence J., and Ian Gold
  2012 Re-Socializing Psychiatry: Critical Neuroscience and the Limits of Reductionism.
    In *Critical Neuroscience: A Handbook of the Social and Cultural Contexts of
    Neuroscience*. J. S. Suparna Choudhury, ed. Pp. 305–30. Oxford, UK: Wiley-
    Blackwell.

Kleinman, Arthur
  1980 *Patients and Healers in the Context of Culture: An Exploration of the Borderland
    Between Anthropology, Medicine, and Psychiatry*. Volume 3. Los Angeles: University
    of California Press.
  1999a Experience and Its Moral Modes: Culture, Human Conditions, and Disorder. In
    The Tanner Lectures on Human Values. G. B. Peterson, ed. Pp. 357–420. Salt Lake
    City: University of Utah Press.
  1999b Moral Experience and Ethical Reflection: Can Ethnography Reconcile Them? A
    Quandary for "The New Bioethics." *Daedalus* Fall 1999.

Kraepelin, Emil
  1902 Dementia Praecox. In *Clinical Psychiatry: A Textbook for Students and Physicians*. E.
    Kraepelin, ed. Pp. 152–202. New York: MacMillan.

Kreyenbuhl, Julie, Ilana R. Nossel, and Lisa B. Dixon
  2009 Disengagement from Mental Health Treatment among Individuals with
    Schizophrenia and Strategies for Facilitating Connections to Care: A Review of the
    Literature. *Schizophrenia Bulletin* 35(4):696–703.

Kruger, Arnold
  2000 Schizophrenia: Recovery And Hope. *Psychiatric Rehabilitation Journal* 24(1):29–37.

Lacro, Jonathan P., L. B. Dunn, C. R. Dolder, S. G. Leckband, and Dilip V. Jeste
  2002 Prevalence of and Risk Factors for Medication Nonadherence in Patients with
    Schizophrenia: A Comprehensive Review of the Literature. *Journal of Clinical
    Psychiatry* 63(10):892–909.

Lear, Jonathan
  2006 *Radical Hope*. Boston, MA: Harvard University Press.

Lewis, Bradley
  2006 A Mad Fight: Psychiatry and Disability Activism. In *The Disability Studies Reader*. L.
    J. Davis, ed. Pp. 339–354. New York: Taylor and Francis.

Lewis, Sara E., Kim Hopper, and Ellen Healion
  2012 Partners in Recovery: Social Support and Accountability in a Consumer-Run
    Mental Health Center. *Psychiatric Services* 63(1):61–65.

Liberman, Robert Paul, and Alex Kopelowicz
  2002 Recovery from Schizophrenia: A Challenge for the 21st Century. *International
    Review of Psychiatry* 14(4):245–55.

Link, Bruce G., Elmer L. Struening, Michael Rahav, Jo C. Phelan, and Larry Nuttbrock
  1997 On Stigma and Its Consequences: Evidence from a Longitudinal Study of Men
    with Dual Diagnoses of Mental Illness and Substance Abuse. *Journal of Health and
    Social Behavior* 38(2):177–90.

Lipsky, Michael
  2010 *Street-Level Bureaucracy: Dilemmas of the Individual in Public Services*. Russell Sage
    Foundation.

Lloyd-Evans, B., M. Crosby, S. Stockton, S. Piling, L. Hobbs, M. Hinton, and S. Johnson

2011 Initiatives to Shorten Duration of Untreated Psychosis: Systematic Review. *British Journal of Psychiatry* 198(4):256–63.

Lloyd-Evans, B., E. Mayo-Wilson, B. Harrison, H. Istead, E. Brown, S. Pilling, S. Johnson, and T. Kendall

2014 A Systematic Review and Meta-Analysis of Randomised Controlled Trials of Peer Support for People with Severe Mental Illness. *BMC Psychiatry* 14(1):39

Locke, John

1823 *An Essay Concerning Human Understanding.* London: Collier Books.

Lord, John, and Francine Dufort

1996 Power and Oppression in Mental Health. *Canadian Journal of Community Mental Health* 15(2):5–22.

Lovell, Anne M.

1997 Narratives of Schizophrenia and Homelessness. *American Anthropologist* 99(2):355–68.

Luhrmann, Tanya M.

2001 *Of Two Minds: The Growing Disorder in American Psychiatry.* New York: Vintage Books.

2007 Social Defeat and the Culture of Chronicity: Or, Why Schizophrenia Does So Well Over There and So Badly Here. *Culture, Medicine, and Psychiatry* 31(2):135–72.

2008 "The Street Will Drive You Crazy": Why Homeless Psychotic Women in the Institutional Circuit in the United States Say No to Offers of Help. *American Journal of Psychiatry* 165(1):15–20.

Marrow, J., and T. M. Luhrmann

2012 The Zone of Social Abandonment in Cultural Geography: On the Street in the United States, inside the Family in India. *Culture, Medicine, and Psychiatry* 36(3):493–513.

Marshall, M., S. Lewis, A. Lockwood, R. Drake, P. Jones, and T. Croudace

2005 Association between Duration of Untreated Psychosis and Outcome in Cohorts of First-Episode Patients: A Systematic Review. *Archives of General Psychiatry* 62(9):975.

McAlpine, Donna D., and Lynn A. Warner

2001 *Barriers to Employment among Persons with Mental Impairments.* New Brunswick, NJ: Institute for Health, Health Care Policy and Aging Research.

McCubbin, Michael

2001 Pathways to Health, Illness and Well-Being: From the Perspective of Power and Control. *Journal of Community & Applied Social Psychology* 11(2):75–81.

McGorry, Patrick

2011 Transition to Adulthood: The Critical Period for Pre-emptive, Disease-Modifying Care for Schizophrenia and Related Disorders. *Schizophrenia Bulletin* 37(3):524.

McLean, Athena Helen

2000 From Ex-Patient Alternatives to Consumer Options: Consequences of Consumerism for Psychiatric Consumers and the Ex-Patient Movement. *International Journal of Health Services* 30(4):821–47.

Mead, Sherry, and Mary Ellen Copeland

2000   What Recovery Means to Us: Consumers' Perspectives. *Community Mental Health Journal* 36(3):315–29.

Mead, Sherry, and David Hilton

2003   Crisis and Connection. *Psychiatric Rehabilitation Journal* 27(1):87–94.

Medscape

2005   An Empowerment Model of Recovery from Severe Mental Illness: An Expert Interview with Daniel B. Fisher. Medscape News & Perspective. *www.medscape. com/viewarticle/496394*.

Mental Health "Recovery" Study Working Group

2009   *Mental Health "Recovery": Users and Refusers.* Toronto: Wellesley Institute.

Metzl, Jonathan M.

2010   *The Protest Psychosis: How Schizophrenia Became a Black Disease.* Boston: Beacon Press.

Mol, Annemarie

2008   *The Logic of Care: Health and the Problem of Patient Choice.* New York: Routledge.

Monahan, John H., H. Steadman, E. Silver, P. Applebaum, P. Robbins, E. Mulvey, L. Roth, T. Grisso, and S. Banks

2001   *Rethinking Risk Assessment: The MacArthur Study of Mental Disorder and Violence.* New York: Oxford University Press.

Mowbray, Carol T., S. P. Moxley, S. Thrasher, D. Bybee, N. McCrohan, S. Harris, and G. Clover

1996   Consumers as Community Support Providers: Issues Created by Role Innovation. *Community Mental Health Journal* 32(1):47–68.

Mowbray, Carol T., Elizabeth A. R. Robinson, and Mark C. Holter

2002   Consumer Drop-In Centers: Operations, Services, and Consumer Involvement. *Health and Social Work* 27(4):248–61.

Mueser, Kim T., Melanie Bennett. and Matthew G. Kushner

1995   Epidemiology of Substance Use Disorders among Persons with Chronic Mental Illnesses. In *Double Jeopardy: Chronic Mental Illness and Substance Use Disorders.* A. Lehman and L. Dixon, eds. Newark, NJ: Harwood Academic.

Mueser, Kim T., Patrick W. Corrigan, David W. Hilton, Beth Tanzman, Annette Schaub, Susan Gingerich, Susan M. Essock, Nick Tarrier, Bodie Morey, Suzanne Vogel-Scibilia, and Marvin I. Herz

2002   Illness Management and Recovery: A Review of the Research. *Psychiatric Services* 53(10):1272–85.

Murphy, Tom

2005   States Crimp Zyprexa Access: Medicaid Restrictions Cutting into Sales of Lilly's Top Drug. *Indianapolis Business Journal* (Nov. 28). *www.ibj.com/articles/17989-states-crimp-zyprexa-access-medicaid-restrictions-cutting-into-sales-of-lilly-s-top-drug*.

Myrdal, Gunnar

1963   *Challenge to Affluence.* New York: Pantheon.

Nelson, Geoffrey, John Lord, and Joanna Ochocka

2001   Empowerment and Mental Health in Community: Narratives of Psychiatric Consumer/Survivors. *Journal of Community & Applied Social Psychology* 11(2):125–42.

North, Carol S.

1987   *Welcome, Silence: My Triumph Over Schizophrenia*. New York: Simon & Schuster.

Nudel, Cassandra

2009   *Firewalkers: Madness, Beauty and Mystery*. Charlottesville, VA: VOCAL.

Nussbaum, Martha C.

2006   *Frontiers of Justice: Disability, Nationality, Species Membership*. London, England: Harvard University Press.

NYOMH, New York State Office of Mental Health

2009   Personalized Recovery Oriented Services. *www.omh.gov/omhweb/pros*.

O'Day, Bonnie, and Mary Killeen

2002   Does US Federal Policy Support Employment and Recovery for People with Psychiatric Disabilities? *Behavioral Sciences & the Law* 20(6):559–83.

Pangle, Lorraine Smith

2007   *The Political Philosophy of Benjamin Franklin*. Baltimore: Johns Hopkins University Press.

Pescosolido, Bernice A., J. K. Martin, and Bruce G. Link

2000   *Americans' Views on Mental Health and Illness at Century's End: Continuity and Change*. Public Report on the MacArthur Mental Health Module, 1996 General Social Survey. Bloomington: Indiana Consortium for Mental Health Services Research, Indiana University and Joseph P. Mailman School of Public Health, Columbia University.

Pierce, Russell D.

2004   A Narrative of Hope. *Psychiatric Rehabilitation Journal* 27(4):403–9.

Pitt, Veronica Jean, Dianne Lowe, Megan Prictor, Sarah Hetrick, Rebecca Ryan, Lynda Berends, and Sophie Hill

2013   A Systematic Review of Consumer-Providers' Effects on Client Outcomes in Statutory Mental Health Services: The Evidence and the Path Beyond. *Journal of the Society for Social Work and Research* 4(4):333–56.

PNFCMH, President's New Freedom Commission on Mental Health

2003   *Achieving the Promise: Transforming Mental Health Care in America*. Pub. SMA03-3831. Rockville, MD: Author. *govinfo.library.unt.edu/mentalhealthcommission/reports/FinalReport/downloads/downloads.html*.

Porter, Roy

2002   *Madness: A Brief History*. London: Oxford University Press.

Pyke, Jennifer, Janis Lancaster, and Jane Pritchard

1997   Training for Partnership. *Psychiatric Rehabilitation Journal* 21(1):64–66.

Rabinow, Paul

1977   *Reflections on Fieldwork in Morocco*. Los Angeles: University of California Press.

Ragins, Mark

2002   A Guide to Mental Health Transformation on a Personal Level. *mhavillage. squarespace.com/section5/2011/12/6/a-guide-to-mental-health-transformation-on-a-personal-level.html*.

Rapp, Charles A.

1998   *The Strengths Model: Case Management with Persons Suffering from Severe and Persistent Mental Illness*. New York: Oxford.

Reno, Virginia P., Jerry L. Mashaw, and Bill Gradison

1997 *Disability: Challenges for Social Insurance, Health Care Financing and Labor Market Policy.* Washington, DC: National Academy of Social Insurance.

Rhodes, Lorna A.

1991 *Emptying Beds: The Work of an Emergency Psychiatric Unit.* Los Angeles: University of California Press.

Ridgway, Priscilla, Diane McDiarmid, Lori Davidson, Julie Bayes, and Sarah Ratzlaff

2002 *Pathways to Recovery: A Strengths Recovery Self Help Workbook.* Auburn Hills, MI: Data Production Corporation.

Rissmiller, David J., and Joshua H. Rissmiller

2006 Evolution of the Antipsychiatry Movement into Mental Health Consumerism. *Psychiatric Services* 57(6):863–66.

Romme, Marius

2000 *Understanding Voices: Coping with Auditory Hallucinations and Confusing Realities.* Gloucester, UK: Handsell Publishing.

Romme, Marius, and Sandra Escher

1989 Hearing Voices. *Schizophrenia Bulletin* 15(2):209–16.

Romme, Marius, Sandra Escher, Jacqui Dillon, Dirk Corstens, and Mervyn Morris

2009 *Living with Voices: 50 Stories of Recovery.* Gateshead, UK: Athaeneum Press.

Rowe, Michael, Jennifer Fret, Margaret Bailey, Deborah Fisk, and Larry Davidson

2001 Clinical Responsibility and Client Autonomy: Dilemmas in Mental Health Work at the Margins. *American Journal of Orthopsychiatry* 71(2):400–407.

Rush, Benjamin

1786 An Inquiry into the Influence of Physical Causes upon the Moral Faculty. In *Medical Inquiries and Observations.* B. Rush, ed. Pp. 93–124. Philadelphia: Carey.

1830 *Medical Inquiries and Observations upon the Diseases of the Mind.* Philadelphia: Grigg.

Rutman, Irvin D.

1994 How Psychiatric Disability Expresses Itself as a Barrier to Employment. *Psychosocial Rehabilitation Journal* 17(3):15–35.

Saez, Mari Almudena, Ann Kelly, and Hannah Brown

2014 Notes from Case Zero: Anthropology in the Time of Ebola. Blog post, September 14. Somatosphere. *somatosphere.net/2014/09/notes-from-case-zero-anthropology-in-the-time-of-ebola.html.*

Saks, Elyn

2007 *The Center Cannot Hold: My Journey through Madness.* New York: Hyperion.

Salzer, Mark, Edward Schwenk, and Eugene Brusilovskiy

2010 Certified Peer Specialist Roles and Activities: Results from a National Survey. *Psychiatric Services* 61(5):520–23.

SAMHSA, Substance Abuse and Mental Health Services Administration

2006 *National Consensus Statement on Mental Health Recovery.* Washington, DC: US Department of Health and Human Servics, Substance Abuse and Mental Health Services Administration, Center for Mental Health Services.

Sayce, Liz

2000 *From Psychiatric Patient to Citizen: Overcoming Discrimination and Social Exclusion.* New York: St Martin's Press.

Schecter, E. S.

1997   Work While Receiving Disability Insurance Benefits: Additional Findings from the New Beneficiary Follow-up Survey. *Social Security Bulletin* 60(1):3–17.

Schiff, Anna Coodin

2004   Recovery and Mental Illness: Analysis and Personal Reflections. *Psychiatric Rehabilitation Journal* 27(3):212–18.

Schiller, Lori, and Amanda Bennet

1996   *The Quiet Room: A Journey Out of the Torment of Madness*. Warner Books Edition: New York.

Schizophrenia.com

2005   Joseph Rogers Success Story. Blog post, May 2. *Schizophrenia Daily News*. *www.schizophrenia.com/sznews/archives/001730.html.*

Schutt, R. K., and E. S. Rogers

2009   Empowerment and Peer Support: Structure and Process of Self Help in a Consumer Run Center for Individuals with Mental Illness. *Journal of Community Psychology* 37(6):697–710.

Segal, Steven P., Carol Silverman, and Tanya Temkin

1995   Measuring Empowerment in Client-Run Self-Help Agencies. *Community Mental Health Journal* 31(3):215–27.

Sells, David J., David A. Stayner, and Larry Davidson

2004   Recovering the Self in Schizophrenia: An Integrative Review of Qualitative Studies. *Psychiatric Quarterly* 75(1):87–96.

Sheitman, Brian B., and Jeffrey A. Lieberman

1998   The Natural History and Pathophysiology of Treatment Resistant Schizophrenia. *Journal of Psychiatric Research* 32(3/4):143–50.

Shorter, Edward

1997   *A History of Psychiatry: From the Era of Asylum to the Age of Prozac*. New York: John Wiley & Sons, Inc.

Smith, Adam

1904   [1776] *An Inquiry into the Nature and Causes of the Wealth of Nations*. London: Methuen and Co.

Smith, Mieko Kotake

2000   Recovery From a Severe Psychiatric Disability: Findings of a Qualitative Study. *Psychiatric Rehabilitation Journal* 24(2):149–58.

Solomon, Phyllis, and Jeffrey Draine

1996   Perspectives Concerning Consumers as Case Managers. *Community Mental Health Journal* 32(1):41–47.

2001   The State Knowledge of the Effectiveness of Consumer Provided Services. *Psychiatric Rehabilitation Journal* 25(1):20–28.

Solomon, Phyllis, and Victoria Stanhope

2004   Recovery: Expanding the Vision of Evidence-Based Practice. *Brief Treatment and Crisis Intervention* 4(4):311–21.

Spaniol, Leroy, Nancy J. Wewiorski, Cheryl Gagne, and William A. Anthony

2002   The Process of Recovery from Schizophrenia. *International Review of Psychiatry* 14(4):327–36.

Steadman, Henry J., F. Osher, P. C. Robbins, B. Case, and S. Samuels
2009   Prevalence of Serious Mental Illness Among Jail Inmates. *Psychiatric Services* 60(6):761–65.

Steele, Ken, and Claire Berman
2001   *The Day the Voices Stopped*. New York: Basic Books.

Stefan, Susan
2002   "Discredited" and "Discreditable": The Search for Political Identity by People with Psychiatric Diagnoses. *William and Mary Law Review* 44:1341–83.

Swarbrick, Margaret
2007   Consumer-Operated Self-Help Centers. *Psychiatric Rehabilitation Journal* 31(1):76–79.

Tanenbaum, Sandra
2011   Mental Health Consumer-Operated Services Organizations in the US: Citizenship as a Core Function and Strategy for Growth. *Health Care Analysis* 19:192–205.

Teplin, Linda A., Gary M. McClelland, Karen M. Abram, and Dana A. Weiner
2005   Crime Victimization in Adults with Severe Mental Illness: Comparison with the National Crime Victimization Survey. *Archives of General Psychiatry* 62(8):911–21.

Tocqueville, Alexis de
2000   [1840] *Democracy in America*. II. Mansfield and D. Winthrop, transl. Chicago: University of Chicago Press.

Tomes, Nancy
1984   *A Generous Confidence: Thomas Story Kirkbride and the Art of Asylum-Keeping, 1840–1883*. London: Cambridge University Press.

Torgalsboen, Anne-Kari
2005   What is Recovery in Schizophrenia? In *Recovery from Severe Mental Illness: Research Evidence and Implications for Practice*. L. Davidson, C. Harding, and L. Spaniol, eds. Pp. 302–15. Boston, Mass: Center for Psychiatric Rehabilitation, Sargent College of Health and Rehabilitation Sciences, Boston University.

Torrey, E. Fuller
1997   *Out of the Shadows: Confronting America's Mental Illness Crisis*. New York: Wiley.

Tsai, Alice
2002   The Story of My Recovery. *Psychiatric Rehabilitation Journal* 25(3):314–15.

Twain, Mark
2002   [1885] *Adventures of Huckleberry Finn*. New York: Penguin Classics.

Van Tosh, Laura
1993   *Working for a Change: Employment of Consumers/Survivors in the Design and Provision of Services for Persons Who are Homeless and Mentally Disabled*. Rockville, MD: Center for Mental Health Services.

Veysey, Bonita, Henry J. Steadman, Joseph P. Morrissey, and Matthew Johnsen
1997   In Search of the Missing Linkages: Continuity of Care in US Jails. *Behavioral Sciences & the Law* 15(4):383–97.

Walsh, Dale
1996   A Journey Toward Recovery: From the Inside Out. *Psychiatric Rehabilitation Journal* 20(2):85–89.

Walsh, Joseph
2000 *Clinical Case Management with Persons Having Mental Illness.* Canada: Wadsworth Thomson Learning.
Wang, Philip S., Olga Demler, and Ronald C. Kessler
2002 Adequacy of Treatment for Serious Mental Disorders in the United States. *American Journal of Public Health* 92(1):92–98.
Ware, Norma C., Kim Hopper, Toni Tugenberg, Barbara Dickey, and D. Fisher
2007 Connectedness and Citizenship. *Psychiatric Services* 58(4):469–75.
Ware, Norma C., Toni Tugenberg, and Barbara Dickey
2004 Practitioner Relationships and Quality of Care for Low-Income Persons with Serious Mental Illness. *Psychiatric Services* 55(5):555–59.
Ware, Norma C., Kim Hopper, Toni Tugenberg, Barbara Dickey, and D. Fisher
2008 A Theory of Social Integration as Quality of Life. *Psychiatric Services* 59(1):27–33.
Warner, Richard
2004 *Recovery from Schizophrenia: Psychiatry and Political Economy.* London: Brunner-Routledge.
Weber, Max
1930 *The Protestant Ethic and the Spirit of Capitalism.* T. Parsons, transl. New York: Routledge.
West, C.
2011 Powerful Choices: Peer Support and Individualized Medication Self-Determination. *Schizophrenia Bulletin* 37(3):445.
Wiseman, Jacqueline P.
1979 *Stations of the Lost: The Treatment of Skid Row Alcoholics.* University of Chicago Press.
Wright, Anthony G.
2012 Social Defeat in Recovery-Oriented Supported Housing: Moral Experience, Stigma, and Ideological Resistance. *Culture, Medicine, and Psychiatry* 36(4):660–78.
Zinman, Sally, Howie T. Harp, and Su Budd
1987 *Reaching Across: Mental Health Clients Helping Each Other.* Riverside, CA: California Network of Mental Health Clients.

INDEX

social dignity, 135
Social Security Amendments (1965), 37
Social Security Disability Insurance
    (SSDI), 17
solidarity, 135
Steve (Horizons' CEO), 2, 8–10, 37, 54,
    89
stigma, 66, 73
substance abuse, 40–41, 76–79
Supplemental Security Income (SSI), 17,
    150
surveillance, 98

tardive dyskinesia, 57–58, 71, 73
Thelma (peer provider), 62–65, 127
This American Life (National Public Radio
    show), 52
Thorazine (chlorpromazine), 67
Tocqueville, Alexis de, 167n4, 168n3
Tony (member), 76
Trey (member), 146
Twain, Mark, 52

US Food and Drug Administration
    (FDA), 67

Vera (peer provider)
    on anger, 144
    Business Center and, 113
    clinical boundaries and, 133–34
    "eating anywhere" and, 110–12, 115–18
    on empowerment and freedom, 87,
        110
    history of, 30–31

medical leave and, 142
medications and, 1, 73–76, 79, 84
neighbors and, 51
newcomers and, 15–16, 29–30, 42–43,
    138
nursing homes and, 36–37, 150–52
on peer providers, 11, 149–50
PEP Members' Council and, 114–16
radical hope and, 153–54
recovery model and, 9–10
Recovery Steering Committee and,
    108
relationships and, 138–39
self-advocacy and, 109–10
on work, 1–2, 52–53, 125
See also Peer Empowerment Program
    (PEP)
Vermont Longitudinal Study, 4–5
violent crime, 66
Vlad (member), 35, 39, 125

Wade (member), 105–6
warming centers, 32
Weber, Max, 54
Wellness Recovery Action Program
    (WRAP), 160
Will (member), 31–32
work
    as challenge, 23–26
    recovery model and, 1–2, 52–55, 76,
        121–29, 147–50

Zyprexa, 18